The Eradication of Dracunculiasis (Guinea Worm Disease) in Nigeria

The Eradication of Dracunculiasis (Guinea Worm Disease) in Nigeria

An Eyewitness Account

LUKE EKUNDAYO EDUNGBOLA, PHD
The Johns Hopkins

ELSEVIER

ELSEVIER

Academic Press is an imprint of Elsevier
125 London Wall, London EC2Y 5AS, United Kingdom
525 B Street, Suite 1650, San Diego, CA 92101, United States
50 Hampshire Street, 5th Floor, Cambridge, MA 02139, United States
The Boulevard, Langford Lane, Kidlington, Oxford OX5 1GB, United Kingdom

The Eradication of Dracunculiasis (Guinea Worm Disease) in Nigeria   ISBN: 978-0-12-816764-9

Publisher: John Fedor
Acquisition Editor: Linda Versteeg-buschman
Editorial Project Manager: Tracy I. Tufaga
Production Project Manager: Kiruthika Govindaraju
Cover Designer: Miles Hitchen

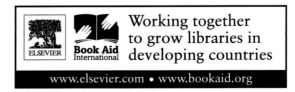

Dedication

I joyfully, responsibly, justifiably, and wholeheartedly dedicate this book to:

1. General Ibrahim B. Babangida, GCFR (former President of Nigeria);

2. President Jimmy and Mrs. Rosalynn Carter (the 39th President of the United States of America and the Chairman of The Carter Center);

3. Gen. Dr. Yakubu Gowon (Nigeria's former Head of State and Chairman, Yakubu Gowon Centre);

4. Mr. Richard Reid (former UNICEF Country Representative in Nigeria);

5. Dr. Donald R. Hopkins (Vice-President and Director of Health Programs, The Carter Center, Atlanta, GA, USA) and

6. The late Professor Olikoye Ransome-Kuti (former Hon. Minister of Health, Nigeria).

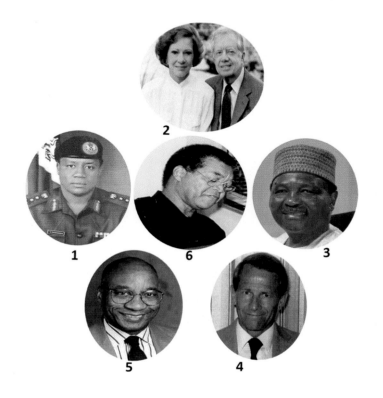

Contents

APPENDICES

Front Cover Photograph

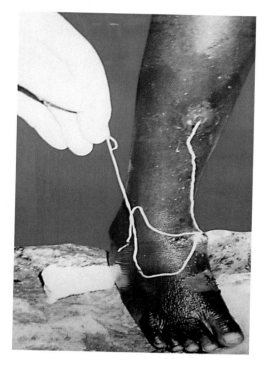

Right leg of a young house-wife showing two protruding adult female *Dracunculus medinensis* (guinea worm).

Foreword

Guinea worm disease (dracunculiasis), has afflicted humans for thousands of years and calcified worms have been identified in Egyptian mummies. Over the years, there were sporadic records of the infection by travelers in West Africa and in articles in scientific journals but little was done to redress the situation. Professor Luke Edungbola played a major role in initiating, organizing, and publicizing the first ever National Conference on Dracunculiasis in Nigeria and in Africa. This was held in 1985 in Kwara Hotel Ilorin, Kwara State, Nigeria. The aim of the conference was to 'bring together many individuals who are interested in this disease in order to assess, in a comprehensive manner, the extent of its problem and what to do about it.'

The conference which was sponsored by the Federal Ministry of Health, the United Nations Children's Fund (UNICEF), the World Health Organization (WHO) and the University of Ilorin, in collaboration with the US Centers for Disease Control and Prevention, brought this neglected and previously almost invisible water-related disease to national and international attention with a determined focus on the urgency to eliminate it as an avoidable cause of unnecessary suffering, protracted incapacitation, impoverishment, underdevelopment and even death, especially when complicated by secondary bacterial infections.

Ironically, the victims of Guinea worm disease are highly disadvantaged, remote, poor rural dwellers with no safe drinking water and who are ignorant of how it is transmitted and can be prevented.

This book is a first-hand account of the many activities that followed the 1985 conference and the establishment of the Nigeria Guinea Worm Eradication Programme (NIGEP), with the challenging mandate to lead the elimination of Guinea worm disease in Nigeria. At the onset, Nigeria had the highest number of dracunculiasis cases in the World.

This book authoritatively and factually presents what Guinea worm disease is, its historical account, its mode of transmission, its impact, the establishment of NIGEP and the intervention strategies adopted by NIGEP to eliminate the disease, in collaboration with The Carter Center, UNICEF, WHO, the United Nations Development Programme and other international partners. This book contains several thrilling, informative, instructive, gruesome and heartbreaking encounters of the 25-year battle that led to the elimination of Guinea worm disease in Nigeria.

The challenges encountered and the gains and benefits that accrued from the successful elimination of the disease are well documented and made relevant to the global control or eradication of other tropical diseases.

The public health community at large and especially those who have been privileged over the years to work with Professor Edungbola on this project, acknowledge his energy, enthusiasm, dedication and sacrifices to the keynote theme of the 1985 conference. "Safe water — the key to good health." We can now rejoice that Guinea worm disease is no longer a threat to livelihoods and health.

During my time at the Department of Geography at the University of Ilorin, I had the privilege of working with Professor Edungbola while we were documenting Guinea worm disease in villages in Kwara State and its environs.

The conclusion in this book is unique, attributing the successful elimination of dracunculiasis in Nigeria to multiple factors but, most strikingly, identifying the most effective of all the intervention strategies used. It is intriguing that the most effective strategy identified could be used not only for the eradication of Guinea worm disease but also for the control and/or eradication of other tropical diseases and conditions.

The book ends with some very memorable and fascinating appendices, including the list of key stakeholders who were involved in the dramatic elimination of Guinea worm disease in Nigeria and the unprecedented postage stamps commemorating Guinea worm disease.

Excluding the appendices, this book contains some 20 assorted, challenging, inspiring, revealing and historical accounts of dracunculiasis, all beautifully illustrated with striking photographs and tables.

This book is a most current, comprehensive, first of its kind on Guinea worm disease and written by an experienced Professor of Medical and Public Health Parasitology, a leading pioneer of dracunculiasis elimination in Nigeria, a Senior Consultant with Global 2000/The Carter Center on dracunculiasis for 25 years, and an eyewitness of the establishment of NIGEP and the implementation of intervention strategies that led to the elimination of Guinea worm disease in Nigeria.

I strongly recommend the book to a wide audience, including medical, paramedical and public health professionals. The book will also be most useful for postgraduate and undergraduate programs in life sciences, community health officers' programs, schools of health technology, nursing, health education, students of arts and culture, mass communication, integrated curricula and medical history.

The book will be valuable in libraries and benefit programs, activities and the services of community and religious leaders, politicians, the United Nations and non-government organizations.

Therefore, regardless of professions, positions, and circumstances, I strongly recommend this excellent, informative, and unique eyewitness account of the elimination of Guinea worm disease in Nigeria to all.

Dr. Susan J. Watts
Former Senior Lecturer at the University of Ilorin, Nigeria
Senior Research Associates (American University in Cairo)
Social Scientist (WHO EMRO)

Preface

In response to launching the target of the First International Drinking Water and Sanitation Decade (1981—91) and in compliance to the implementation of the World Health Assembly Resolution (WHA 39.21), which called for the eradication of dracunculiasis (Guinea worm disease), the First National Conference on Dracunculiasis in Nigeria (and in Africa) was held in Ilorin, Kwara State, Nigeria, from March 23 to 25, 1985. The conference heralded the beginning of concerted efforts to raise public and political awareness of the occurrence, magnitude, impact and spread of Guinea worm disease in the country (for the first time) and the urgency of launching effective interventions.

Thereafter, the Federal Government of Nigeria signed a Memorandum of Understanding with Global 2000/The Carter Center for the elimination of Guinea worm disease in Nigeria. The Nigeria Guinea Worm Eradication Program (NIGEP) was also inaugurated with the mandate to spearhead activities that would lead to the elimination of this ancient water-transmitted, very debilitating and very impoverishing disease in Nigeria.

The zoning structure of the four Primary Health Care system was to be used as the operational basis nationwide, adopting safe water supply, health education, vector control (using temephos [Abate]) and water filtration (using nylon monofilament filters) as the core national strategies.

The late Professor Olikoye Ransome-Kuti, Nigeria's Honorable Minister of Health, played a most active role in the establishment and operation of NIGEP, in the co-sponsoring of eradication of dracunculiasis at the 39th WHA and in the signing of the Memorandum of Understanding with The Carter Center, under the Chairmanship of the former American President, Hon. Jimmy Carter, on behalf of the Federal Government.

The initial challenges confronting NIGEP were the non-availability of reliable data on the spread and magnitude of the dracunculiasis problem in the country, on the knowledge, attitude, and practices of the multi-ethnic and highly diversified populations socioculturally and on the impact assessment of the disease which was necessary to promote advocacy, community mobilization, public enlightenment, planning and to solicit for international partnership and support.

In the first Active Case Search conducted in 1987/1988 (July 01 to June 30) a staggering number of about 700,000 cases of Guinea worm disease in some 6000 endemic villages were recorded. Thus, Nigeria was ranked as the most endemic country in the world. This, with the relatively huge size of Nigeria, highly diversified ethnicity, about 70% rural population (many inaccessible and "at the end of the road") and relative political instability, there was global skepticism that if Nigeria could eliminate her Guinea worm disease at all, she would be the last country in the world to do so.

Ironically, through very strong and consistent political commitment, good program structures and implementation, and strong international support (The Carter Center, United Nations Children's Fund, World Health Organization, United Nations Development Programme, Japan International Cooperation Agency, etc.), Nigeria stunned the world when the World Health Organization certified Nigeria free of dracunculiasis in 2013!

This book, written by a leading pioneer of dracunculiasis elimination in Nigeria for about 35 years and a Senior Consultant to Global 2000/The Carter Center for about 25 years presents an authoritative, factual and most current eye-witness account of the elimination of Guinea worm disease in Nigeria, using his wealth of experiences in the North West Zone (eight States and the Federal Capital Territory, Abuja). Strikingly, the zone had the two mixed types of transmissions (raining and dry season types) found in Nigeria.

The book succinctly highlights the implementation of various core and supportive strategies adopted for the elimination of Guinea worm disease in Nigeria.

The book features: a wide range of original topics; fascinating personal and collective encounters; what Guinea worm disease is; the transmission and impact of the disease; the epidemiology and historical account of the disease; the structure and strategies of NIGEP; the trends of Guinea worm disease elimination in Nigeria over a period of 25 years (1988—2013); several horrifying and dramatic experiences; the justification, feasibility and challenges of dracunculiasis elimination; lessons, gains and benefits of Guinea worm disease elimination and the global relevance of the experiences acquired during Guinea worm disease elimination to combating other tropical diseases.

The issue of program stagnation, some 20 phenomenal but real-life experiences, multiple gruesome encounters, unique memorable events, blessings even in uncommon circumstances, and the fate of the fountain pen donated to sign the obituary of Guinea worm disease are all well-documented topics that must be read.

In conclusion, the book enumerates the trials, tribulations, challenges and scars of the battle to eliminate Guinea worm disease as a public health problem. It asserts that the end has justified the means after a 25-year battle to eliminate the disease. The book also identifies the most potent and decisive of all the interventions used for the elimination of dracunculiasis and potentially for other tropical diseases.

The book ends with six richly illustrated appendices: logos of some key stakeholders and partners; Nigeria's Guinea worm disease commemorative postage stamps; Some Memorable Notes on Dracunculiasis from Friends/Colleagues; the Guinea worm race; memorable photographs during Guinea worm disease elimination

activities and quotable quotes on Guinea worm disease. Similarly, the book presents world records of the man with the highest number of emerging adult female Guinea worms (84) on his body during a single transmission year and the woman with 62 emerging worms.

This book, in its own way, is original, factual, thrilling, fascinating, entertaining, revealing, informative, educative, challenging, inspiring, historical and richly illustrated.

Some previously undocumented information relevant to dracunculiasis eradication is presented in this book. The book uses the experience of dracunculiasis elimination in Nigeria as a case model for effective interventions against other tropical diseases.

The most notable and ultimate lesson of the elimination of Guinea worm disease in Nigeria, as documented in this book, is the dramatic transformation from pain, poverty and neglect to prosperity, happiness, and celebrations of wellness and productive lives.

The contents of this book are by no means exhaustive or exactly chronological. However, they are unequivocally authentic and factual to the best of human recall, judgment and packaging.

Luke Ekundayo Edungbola, PhD
The Johns Hopkins

Acknowledgments

One of my greatest problems in writing this book is how to express my profound gratitude to so many deserving individuals, groups and organizations.

However, in view of the considerable demands, challenges and personal encounters that I experienced during my 35 years of active participation in dracunculiasis elimination in Nigeria and elsewhere, I am most grateful to the Almighty God who made "The End to Justify the Means". "Many, Lord our God, are the wonders You have done", the eradication of dracunculiasis is one of them!

I am highly indebted to all who, in one way or the other, supported me, prayed for me, sponsored me, and contributed positively to my role in the elimination of Guinea worm disease in Nigeria. The endless list includes: The Carter Center; the United Nations Children's Fund (UNICEF); the World Health Organization (WHO); The United Nations Development Programme; Federal, State and Local Government Areas; Professor Olikoye Ransome-Kuti (former Hon. Minister of Health); former American president, President Jimmy and Mrs. Rosalynn Carter; Gen. Dr. Yakubu Gowon (former Nigerian Head of State); President General Ibrahim B. Babangida (GCFR); Late President Umaru Yar'Adua; Professor A.B.C. Nwosu (former Minister of Health); Professor Eyitayo Lambo (former Minister of Health); His Excellency Alh. Aliyu Magatakarda Wamakko (former Governor of Sokoto State); His Excellency, Late Prince Audu Abubakar (former Governor of Kogi State); Chief Cornelius O. Adebayo (Former Governor of Kwara State); Group Captain Salaudeen A. Latinwo (former Military Governor of Kwara State); Group Captain Ibrahim Alkali (former Military Governor of Kwara State); Colonel Alwali I. Kazir (former Military Governor of Kwara State); Dr. Bukola Saraki (former Governor of Kwara State); Governor Abdulfatai Ahmed (Governor of Kwara State); Alh. Senator Tijani Yahaha (the Tafida of Kaura and former Chairman of Kaura Namoda Local Government Areas); Mr. Richard Reid (former UNICEF Country Representative, Nigeria), Dr. Donald R. Hopkins (Vice-President and Director of Health programs, The Carter Center, Atlanta, GA); Mr. David Bassiouni (UNICEF Senior Program Officer) and Dr. Carel de Roy (UNICEF-Water and Sanitation, Nigeria).

I thank The Carter Center Technical Advisers in Nigeria: Craig Withers, Jr.; Pat McConoor; Mike Street; the late Wayne Duncan and Dr. E.S. Miri (Country Representative for Nigeria) for their support and cooperation.

The NIGEP National Coordinators performed creditably and they are: Dr. Mrs. Lola K. Sadiq; Dr. Mrs. O.O. Ojo; Dr. Mrs. A. Adeyemi; the late Dr. K.A. Ojodu and Dr. Mrs. I.N. Anagbogu.

I thank Professor A.B.O.O. Oyediran (Chairman, National Certification Committee on Guinea Worm Disease Eradication (NCC GWDE) and members of his committee as well as the non-statutory members) for successfully presenting Nigeria to the WHO for Guinea worm disease-free certification.

It was most fulfilling working with my colleagues, the Zonal Facilitators/Senior Zonal Consultants: Professor O.O. Kale; Professor E.I. Braide; Dr. J.O. Ologe; Professor M.K.O. Padonu; Dr. Ben Nwobi; Dr. A. Osibogun; Dr. C. Ityonzughul; Mrs. Maduka; Dr. Adamu Musa and Dr. Mohammed Jabir.

Representatives of Federal, State and Local Government are "warriors" who fought and eliminated Guinea worm disease in the North West Zone include: the late Dr. J.O. Idowu; H. Abe; Prof. S.K. Odaibo; Prof. & Mrs (Pharm) Kuranga; Late Dr. S. Olumo; B. Dogondaji; H. Bujawa; Dr. M. Quabasiyu; the late L. Ajileye; Dr. M.B. Marafa; Dr. M. Ango; I. Gusau; J. Omonayin; T.O. Alabi; B. Olokun; L. Kolawole and M. Awojobi. Among The NIGEP/The Carter Center Zonal Field Staff, in the North West Zone, who fought gallantly and eliminated Guinea worm disease in the zone and in some other zones are: Solomon Olukade; A. Sayaolu; A.Z. Abdulkadir; S. Toye; M. Atolagbe; W. Ogar; O. Oluwole; B. Ahmed; J.O. Bakare; S. Laleye; L. Olapade; L. Ibrahim; A. Olayinka; I. Sardauna; T. Moneke; B. Durojaye; S. Adelamo; Alh. Sadiq; P. Edafidi; H.O Olajide and A. Halima.

The Directors of the Disease Control, Epidemiological Unit and the Primary Health Care Agency (Dr. Gabi Williams, Dr. D.A. Kolawole, Dr. Sorongbe and the late Dr. Mrs. Aromasodu) provided very sound and effective professional guidance.

The University of Ilorin, Ilorin, and the College of Health Sciences provided all the support, encouragement and understanding that enabled me to function optimally and productively. In that regard, I am grateful to Late Professor S. Afolabi Toye (Vice-Chancellor); Professor Adeoye Adeniyi (Vice-Chancellor); Professor Abdulraheem Oba (Vice-Chancellor); Professor O. Ogunremi (Deputy Vice-Chancellor); Professor Pekun Alausa (Chief Medical Director/Dean); Professor E.H.O. Parry (Dean); Professor John Hamilton; Professor I.O. Oloyede (Vice-Chancellor); Professor O.O. Balogun (VC, FUNAAB); Professor Albert Anjorin and Professor and Professor (Mrs) S.O. Amali (Vice-Chancellor).

My pioneering research team on dracunculiasis provided a solid foundation for the First National Conference on Guinea Worm Disease and its elimination. Members include: O.O. Kayode; D.B. Parakoyi; O.O. Agbede; W.B. Ebomoyi; K.S. Adeyemi; E.I.I. Gemade; A.C. Nwosu; S.J. Watts; E.I. Braide; S.O. Asaolu; T.O. Alabi; Albert Anjorin and the late Professors J.D. Adeniyi and A. Yinka-Dopemu.

Without the active participation and cooperation of all the Zonal Field Managers/Supervisors, the Village-Based Health Workers, Local Government Area and State Guinea worm disease Coordinators, Directors of Primary Health Care, community leaders, security and law enforcement agents and school teachers, among others, dracunculiasis elimination would have remained elusive in Nigeria.

I wholeheartedly thank the secretariat personnel that facilitated the preparation of the manuscript and illustrations of this book - Pelumi Adeyemi, Abubakar Bello, Sanmi Adeyemi, John Oshodi, Mudashiru Giwa, Feranmi Folahan, Raphael Ikpe, Adeoluwa Edungbola, Sunday Edungbola and Toluwani Ayandokun.

The *Sunday Concord* and the Nigeria Television Authority Ilorin (Vickie Olumidi, Adeogun Ajala, Yemi Kuforiji, Bosede Adebayo, Moji Makanjoula, Abiodun Balogun and others) ably demonstrated the valuable and indispensable role which print and electronic media can play in the control of tropical and other diseases.

I thank **Elsevier** for accepting to publish this book timely with great understanding, cooperation, encouragement and as a Hot Topic Title.

Acronyms/Abbreviations

CDC	Centers for Disease Control and Prevention
COBES	Community Based Experience and Services
DFRRI	Directorate of Food Roads and Rural Infrastructure
FCT	Federal Capital Territory
GCFR	Grand Commander of the Federal Republic
ICC	International Certification Commission
ICCDE	International Certification Commission on Dracunculiasis Eradication
ICT	International Certification Team
L1	First larva stage
L2	Second larva stage
L3	Third and infective larva stage
LGA	Local Government Areas
MAMSER	Mass Mobilization for Socio-Economic Recovery
NCCG-WDE	National Certification Committee on Guinea Worm Disease Eradication
NIGEP	Nigeria Guinea Worm Eradication Programme
NTA	Nigeria Television Authority
NYSC	National Youth Service Corps
OCP	Onchocerciasis Control Program
PHC	Primary Health Care
RUWATSAN	Rural Water and Sanitation
UNDP	United Nations Development Program
UNICEF	United Nations International Children Emergency Fund
USAID	United States Agency for International Development
VBHW	Village Based Health Workers
WATSAN	Water and Sanitation
WHA	World Health Assembly
WHO	World Health Organization
YGC	Yakubu Gowon Centre

Definitions

1. Guinea Worm Day in Nigeria (March 20) was established to commemorate the First National Conference on Dracunculiasis in Nigeria and to promote political and public awareness of the necessity for and commitment to eliminating Guinea worm disease in Nigeria.

   Over the years, Guinea Worm Day had featured several major events:

   1. Reports of annual Active Case Searches of 1987/1988, 1988/1989, 1989/1990 and 1990/1991;
   2. The launching of the Donor's Meeting;
   3. The launching of Guinea worm commemorative postage stamps
   4. The launching of the Proceedings of the Guinea Worm Conference as supplements of the *Nigerian Journal of Parasitology* and
   5. The presentation of Jimmy and Rosalynn Carter Awards to deserving Nigerians (Zonal Consultants, Local Government Areas Chairmen and NIGEP Field Staff).

2. A case of Guinea worm disease was defined during the Second African Region Conference on Guinea Worm Disease in Accra, Ghana, in 1988 as "An individual exhibiting a skin lesion or lesions with the emergence of one or more Guinea worm (each individual being counted once in a calendar year e.g., July 01–June 30 during Active Case Search and January 01–December 31 during Active Monthly Surveillance"

3. Lifecycle/Developmental Biology is a sequential but phenomenal event during which a living organism, e.g., a Guinea worm undergoes multiple biological transformations to attain infectivity and maturity

4. Adult/mature parasite is the stage when the parasite is capable of sexual production

5. Target organ is the predestined site in the final host where the matured/adult parasite resides

6. Intermediate or secondary host is the biological agent that harbors the immature parasite and facilitates the biological transformation of a parasite from non-infective to infective stage. The intermediate host for the Guinea worm is *Cyclops* (copepods or water fleas)

7. Final/definite host is the host in which the adult/matured parasite lives; man is the definite/final/primary host for the Guinea worm

8. L1, L2 are larval stages of Guinea worm, which are found in water and in *Cyclops*. These larvae are not infective to man until L2 is biological transformed to L3. Anyone drinking contaminated water harboring *Cyclops* with infective (L3) larva will likely manifest emergence of Guinea worm on the body after an incubation period of about 1 year

9. Incubation period is the time between contact with the infection and manifestation of the disease; the incubation period for Guinea worm is about 12 months

10. Direct lifecycle is the acquisition of a parasitic disease in which no biological agent (arthropods, etc.) plays a role in the transformation of the non-infective to the infective stage of the parasite, e.g., the non-infective egg of *Ascaris sp* becoming infective embryonated egg in the soil.

11. Indirect lifecycle is the developmental biology whereby it is mandatory for a biological agent to facilitate the biological transformation of a noninfective to infective stage of the parasite, e.g., it is only in *Cyclops* that non-infective larvae of Guinea worm can be transformed biologically to the infective stage.

CHAPTER 1

Introduction to Guinea Worm, Guinea Worm Disease and Its Elimination in Nigeria

WHAT IS GUINEA WORM DISEASE?

Dracunculiasis (Guinea worm disease [GWD]) is a painful and crippling infection caused by a parasitic nematode (round worm), with the Latin name *Dracunculiasis medinensis* (Linnaeus 1758, Gallandant 1773).

Dracunculiasis has been known since antiquity, and thus it is known by many vernaculars in different parts of the world and geographic locations where the disease is found. Such names include: Guinea worm; Medina worm; filaire de mediine, le dragonneau and pharaonsurm.[1] Its local tribal names in Nigeria include: Sobia in Yoruba; Kurkunnu in Hausa; Arikwa Mmiri in Igbo; Ngudu in Kanuri; Jigan in Tiv; Otombia in Agatu; Bulutu in Fulani; Sombia in Gwari; Sonbiya in Nupe; Tandu in Baruten; Zuba in Bussa and Tuturiqui in Gwari.

The infection is transmitted to man exclusively by drinking raw (or untreated) stagnant water that has been contaminated by an infected person who immersed a protruding female Guinea worm into the community drinking water source (usually a pond in Nigeria) about 2 weeks previously. Ironically, unlike other human parasites that live in the internal organs (stomach, intestines, livers, lungs, eyes, muscles, brain, red blood cells, macrophages, cerebrospinal fluid, etc.) of their definitive or final hosts (for maximum safety and the supply of essential needs for growth, protection and reproduction), the heavily impregnated but widowed adult female Guinea worm, with thousands of Guinea worm larvae (babies) in her uterus, fearlessly and with outright disregard for the norm, exposes herself by emerging through the human skin, despite the risk involved. This occurs not out of foolishness, daringness or mere parasitic exuberance, but is a mandatory predestined parasitic sacrifice of life (after about a year of living and developing in the human body) to safely discharge thousands of Guinea worm larvae from her uterus into the drinking ponds.

The ultimate intention is to ensure the perpetuation of the species in nature. This is in the spirit of a mother's life for the survival of thousands of her potential offsprings.

The emergence of an adult female Guinea worm through the human skin, after incubating for about a year in the human body, invariably signifies the end of her life span. Unfortunately, this first and last public appearance of the female Guinea worm often leads to severe suffering and pain in the human host. The pains are mostly related to the number and anatomic locations of the emerging worms on the human body and to secondary bacterial infection caused by unhealthy and unsanitary methods of local management, ignorance and taboos. These often prolong incapacitation and lead to severe complications, permanent deformity and even death, especially when associated with tetanus.

For the community at large, in the absence of effective interventions and amid ignorance, repeated multiple infections, poverty and neglect, dracunculiasis often has grave consequences on agriculture, health, education, demography, socioeconomic activities and general development to the extent of impoverishing the entire community year after year.

In endemic areas, multiple infections are rampant. In the North West Zone of the Nigeria Guinea Worm Eradication Programme (NIGEP) where I spearheaded the eradication of dracunculiasis in nine States for more than two decades, a world-record number of 84 worms emerged from a 24-year-old farmer in the Dutsin-Ma Local Government Areas (LGA) of Katsina State in one transmission season (January to December). Among infected females, a maximum of 62 Guinea worms emerged from a housewife in Bungudu LGA of Zamfara State in one transmission period.

All the Guinea worms emerging on the human body are females. The males die in the human host after fertilizing the females, thereby completing their parasitic obligation. Thus, the male Guinea worm never emerges on the human body.

As a parasitic adaptation, more than 90% of adult female Guinea worms emerge on the lower limbs. However, they can emerge at virtually any other anatomic location on the human body, including the breast, scrotum, eyes, head, back, buttocks, hands, fingers, trunk, stomach, and jaw. (Fig. 1.1)

In the endemic areas, dracunculiasis has a negative impact on virtually all aspects of human endeavor, including: agriculture; heath; education; socioeconomics; politics; community development; and the quality of life in general.

Elimination of Dracunculiasis in Nigeria

In response to launching and achieving the targets of the First International Drinking Water and Sanitation Decade (1981−90) and to implementing the World Health Assembly Resolution (WHA 39:21) which called for the eradication of dracunculiasis, the Federal Government of Nigeria inaugurated the NIGEP in 1988. NIGEP's mandate was to spearhead the eradication of GWD in Nigeria, operating in the four Primary Health Care zones and using four core-intervention strategies (safe water supply, health education, vector control with temephos (Abate) and the use of nylon monofilament filters to sieve infected

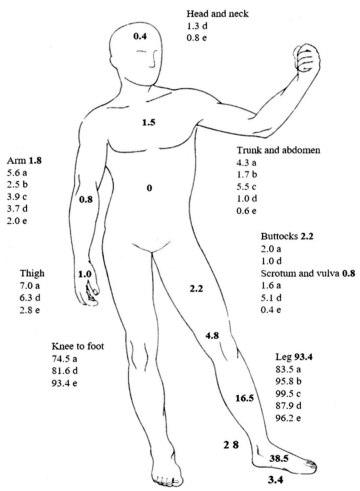

FIG. 1.1 Percentage distribution of guinea worm lesions on the body. Body figures refer to a survey of 267 patients in villages north of Ibadan (Nigeria) in 1967. Other sources: (a) from Fairley (1924); (b) from Lindberg (1946); (C) from Ferreira and Lopes (1948); (d) from Onabamiro (1958); (e) from Rao and Reddy (1965).

cyclops out of the drinking water before consumption). Professor Olikoye Ransome-Kuti, Nigeria's Hon. Minister of Health, played active key roles in the establishment and operation of NIGEP, in co-sponsoring the eradication of dracunculiasis at the 39th WHA and in signing the Memorandum of Understanding for dracunculiasis eradication in Nigeria with The Carter Center under the chairmanship of the former American President, Hon. Jimmy Carter. Dr. Donald R. Hopkins and his Atlanta colleagues were the catalysts and facilitators in Nigeria, as they were for the entire world of dracunculiasis.

NIGEP, with two major national committees (the multisectoral National Task Force and the National Technical Committee), in collaboration with the Federal Government of Nigeria, States and LGAs, enjoyed considerable goodwill, international partnership, and sizable support from The Carter Center, United Nations Children's Fund, World Health Organization (WHO), United Nations Development Programme, Japan International Cooperation Agency and other agencies.

The initial challenge confronting NIGEP was the non-availability of reliable data on the spread and magnitude of the dracunculiasis problem in Nigeria, on the knowledge, attitudes and practices of Nigerians (especially in the endemic areas) and on the impact assessment documentation needed to promote advocacy, community mobilization and public enlightenment and to solicit international support.

The First National Conference on Dracunculiasis in Nigeria (and in Africa) was held in Ilorin, Kwara State, March 23–25, 1985. Participants from Universities, Research Institutes, and from the Federal, State and LGA Ministries of Health, Agriculture, Education, Water Resources, etc., were invited to present any data and information on the status of dracunculiasis in their localities. Resource personnel were invited from the United States (including Centers for Disease Control and Prevention and Global 2000), United Kingdom, India, Onchocerciasis Control Programme and some African countries.

At the end of the conference, using the event as a rapid assessment method to determine the distribution and endemicity of dracunculiasis in Nigeria, an estimated 2.5 million cases of GWD were reported and a map was compiled to document the geographic distribution and endemicity of the disease for the whole country for the first time.[2]

The conference was the beginning of a concerted effort which revealed that GWD was a nationwide problem, occurring in virtually all States and most LGAs. Thereafter, three consecutive active case searches were conducted nationwide between 1988 and 1992. Active monthly surveillance began after the last active case search. Soon after the First National Conference on Dracunculiasis, more concerted studies by researchers began to document the impact of dracunculiasis on agriculture, health, education, sociocultural development and socioeconomic activities.

In 1988, during the Second African Conference on Dracunculiasis in Accra, Ghana, a standard definition of a case of GWD was established for use in all endemic countries:

> *An individual exhibiting a skin lesion or lesions with the emergence of one or more Guinea worm (each individual should be counted once in a calendar year).*

In Nigeria, annual active monthly surveillance began in 1992 from January 01 to December 31, in contrast to active case searching which took place annually between July 01 and June 30.

The first active case search carried out between July 01, 1987 and June 30, 1988, recorded about 700,000 cases of GWD in some 6000 endemic villages nationwide, thus ranking Nigeria as the most endemic country for dracunculiasis in the world.

Global Relevance and Significance of the Elimination of Dracunculiasis in Nigeria

At the onset of the dracunculiasis eradication campaigns and for multiple reasons, there was widespread skepticism that if Nigeria ever eliminated dracunculiasis at all, She would be the last country globally to do so, probably because:

1. of Nigeria's highest number of dracunculiasis cases in the world;
2. the relatively huge size of the country and her highly diversified multi-ethnicity;
3. the challenges of poor accessibility to rural areas "at the end of the road" and
4. the limitations of political will, commitment, stability and corruption.

Ironically, Nigeria stunned the watching world when in 2013, the WHO certified the country free of dracunculiasis following due recommendations by the WHO International Certification Commission.

Before the WHO International Certification Commission's recommendations, Nigeria had recorded zero cases for more than three consecutive years under the monitoring activities of the National Certification Committee on the Eradication of Guinea Worm Disease.

Lessons From the Dracunculiasis Elimination Program

- The elimination of dracunculiasis in Nigeria provides an encouraging and timely impetus for the control and eradication of other tropical diseases if the lessons and strategies used in Nigeria are adopted or modified as required.
- When the campaign for the eradication of dracunculiasis was first launched, there were 3.2 million cases of the disease globally. Thus, today, dracunculiasis eradication is not only very promising but imminent. This breakthrough is a boost for the fight against other tropical diseases after the failure of the malaria eradication campaigns.
- When eradication is achieved, GWD will be the second endemic disease only after smallpox to be eradicated in its natural state. It will also become the first major parasitic disease to be eradicated, strikingly without using drugs or vaccines.
- Although polio eradication is promising, it is a greater challenge because of its epidemiologic phenomenon whereby polio virus can exist in its natural state without evidence of actual cases.
- Unlike polio, with onset of paralytic poliomyelitis after a relatively short incubation period of 1—3 weeks and with more than 70% of polio infections in children asymptomatic,[3] Medina dracunculiasis has an incubation period of about 52 weeks and a well-defined and restricted foci of passive transmissions.

Unlike polio and smallpox eradication, the strategy used for dracunculiasis eradication did not involve the use of any vaccine because there was none.

The core strategies used for the elimination of dracunculiasis in Nigeria were: safe drinking water supply (use and maintenance); continuous and effective health education; the use of nylon monofilament filters (to sieve out infected cyclops from drinking water) and chemical treatment of infected stagnant drinking water sources with temephos (Abate) to kill the cyclops (the exclusive intermediate host for *Dracunculus medinesis*).

Other effective strategies include: case containment; integrated surveillance; cash rewards; investigation of rumored cases and cross-border activities.

In the North West Zone of NIGEP, some radical innovations became very valuable strategies. Such innovations include: large-scale surgical extraction of Guinea worms and case management; the use of pond guards; the introduction of school-based surveillance and the application of the global positioning system to strengthen surveillance documentation.

For the eradication of smallpox, polio and dracunculiasis, massive and continuous health education, effective community mobilization/public enlightenment, strong political will, the active participation of multiple stakeholders, the generous support of international partners, well-monitored surveillance and the adoption of standardized case definitions are common lessons to learn in the fight against tropical diseases.

In the current aspiration, determination, and justification to effectively control and/or eradicate endemic tropical diseases, another significant value to gain from the elimination of dracunculiasis in Nigeria is the prompt timeliness of decisions, actions, and interventions.

If the elimination of GWD in Nigeria had been delayed just for a little while longer, the unfortunate and dramatic emergence, escalation and spread of insurgencies, insecurities, banditry and communal clashes, natural disasters, the magnitude and challenges of managing internally displaced persons, the advent of economic recession, competition for priorities and resources and political will against more deadly diseases, newly emerging diseases, re-emerging diseases and stagnated diseases, would have adversely and tragically prolonged the elimination of dracunculiasis indefinitely, thereby making Nigeria the last country in the world to eliminate dracunculiasis as had been erroneously predicted by many at the onset of the global drive for dracunculiasis eradication.

As is popularly and prayerfully said in Nigeria, "God forbids bad things."

REFERENCES

1. Muller R. In: *Advances in Parasitology*. Vol. 9. London: Academic Press; 1971.
2. Edungbola LD, Watts SJ, Kale OO, Smith GS, Hopkins DR. A method of rapid assessment of the distribution and endemicity of dracunculiasis in Nigeria. *Soc Sci Med*. 1986;23(6): 555—558.
3. Centers for Disease Control and Prevention. Poliomyelitis. In: *Epidemiological and Prevention of Vaccine-Preventable Diseases*. 13th ed.; 2015. Retrieved online https://www.cdc.gov/vaccines/pubs/pinkbook/downloads/polio.pdf.

CHAPTER 2

Transmission, Seasonality and Endemicity of Dracunculiasis

Dracunculiasis cannot be transmitted directly from one person to another. Eating the 1-m-long worm or ingesting thousands of freshly shed larvae cannot lead to the establishment of Guinea worm infection because neither the adult female worm nor her freshly shed L1 larvae are infective to man. For the L1 larvae to become infective to man, they must first be transformed biologically to the infective stage (L3). This transformation can only occur in an appropriate arthropod, a crustacean (*Cyclops* sp.) (Fig. 2.1).

The biological transformation of non-infective larvae (L1 and L2) to infective forms (L3) in cyclops takes about 2 weeks. When the pond water containing cyclops harboring infective larvae (L3) is ingested by man (the final or definitive host), an infection can be established. The victim may not know until after an incubation period of about a year. During the incubation period, the ingested infective male and female larvae grow and mature (capable of mating for production) in the human body.

After about 6 months in the human body, the matured male Guinea worm mates and fertilizes the female. Thereafter, he dies, having successfully accomplished the natural assignment for which he was destined. On the other hand, his female counterpart lives on for another 6 months and by now has thousands of Guinea worm larvae (L1), produced ovoviviparously (eggs hatching to L1 larvae), in her uterus.

After an incubation period of about 12 months, when she is about to emerge through the human skin, the adult female Guinea worm produces a toxin, which elicits tissue necrosis and the formation of blisters. These blisters from which the adult female will emerge can occur on virtually any part of the human body but more than 90% occurs on the lower extremities as a parasitic adaptation (Fig. 2.2A and B).

When these blisters rupture, the female uterus protrudes through the broken blister and when the body part (mostly the lower extremities) bearing the emerging worm is immersed in stagnant water, the drop in temperature causes contraction of the uterus

and the expulsion of hundreds of L1 larvae into the pond. These L1 larvae swim actively, searching for *Cyclops* (intermediate host) in which the L1 will be biologically transformed to infective L3 larvae in about 15 days. Failure of L1 larvae to find appropriate *Cyclops* sp. in time (3 days) will lead to their loss of infectivity and they eventually die.

The knowledge of the mode of transmission of Guinea worms (Fig. 2.3) is fundamental to revealing, understanding and exploiting vulnerable points at which interventions (such as: safe water supply, use, and maintenance; health education; vector control, using temephos (Abate) and water filtration e.g. using nylon monofilament filters) can be effectively targeted for dracunculiasis eradication.

The relatively huge size of Nigeria and the disparities in vegetation and climatic features, affect the transmission, seasonality and endemicity of dracunculiasis throughout the country.

Although the direct effects of climate change on the transmission of Guinea worm disease (GWD) and other tropical diseases have not been fully documented, better understanding of the impact of climate change on disease ecology, in relation to tropical diseases, should constitute a serious public health interest.

Nigeria has two major climatic seasons: the rainy and the dry seasons. Similarly, the vegetation is of two broad varieties, the forest in the south and the savannah in the north.

In the South West and South East, dracunculiasis transmission peaks during the dry season when rivers and streams dry up and form stagnant pools and ponds, becoming a conducive ecological habitat for the breeding of cyclops, the contamination of ponds by infected persons and the transmission of GWD.

In the Northern States, e.g., in the nine States of the Nigeria Guinea Worm Eradication Programme (NIGEP) North West Zone (Fig. 2.4), where I led interventions against dracunculiasis for more than 20 years, the peak transmission is mixed, occurring both during the rainy and dry seasons. Thus, in Sokoto, Zamfara, Kebbi,

The Eradication of Dracunculiasis (Guinea Worm Disease) in Nigeria. https://doi.org/10.1016/B978-0-12-816764-9.00002-X

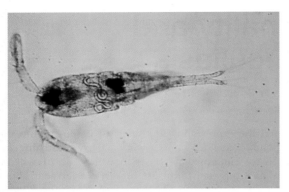

FIG. 2.1 *Cyclops* sp. (Copepod, water fleas) showing Guinea worm larva in the haemocoel of the water fleas. (Source: Ruiz-Tiben and Hopkins (2006).[3])

and Katsina States, the peak transmission occurred during the rainy season (June–October) on the January–December monthly surveillance index. In those States, during the dry season (November–May), water scarcity becomes a major problem. In the desperate search for water, multiple areas were dug out along the dried up river beds and in previously swampy areas. In that process, multiple holes were dug and then abandoned when they no longer yielded water. However, during the rainy season, these abandoned holes were filled with rain water and became stagnant water bodies or ponds, creating a suitable ecological environment for breeding cyclops, contamination by infected persons (while wadding through to fetch water) and the transmission of GWD.

In contrast and in the same NIGEP North West Zone, transmission traditionally peaked during the dry season

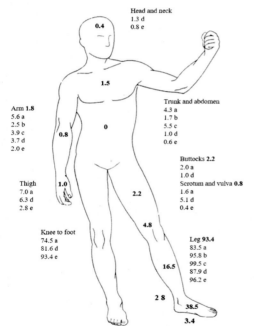

Percentage distribution of guinea worm lesions on the body. Body figures refer to a survey of 267 patients in villages north of Ibadan (Nigeria) in 1967. Other sources: (a) from Fairley (1924); (b) from Lindberg (1946); (C) from Ferreira and Lopes (1948); (d) from Onabamiro (1958); (e) from Rao and Reddy (1965).

A

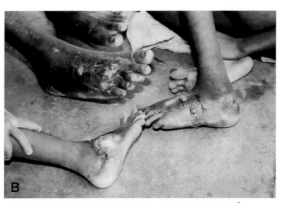

B

FIG. 2.2 **(A)** Sites of emergence of adult female Guinea worms on the human body. (Source: Muller (1971)[5]. **(B)** The lower limbs of school children showing emerging Guinea worms.

Life cycle of the guinea worm

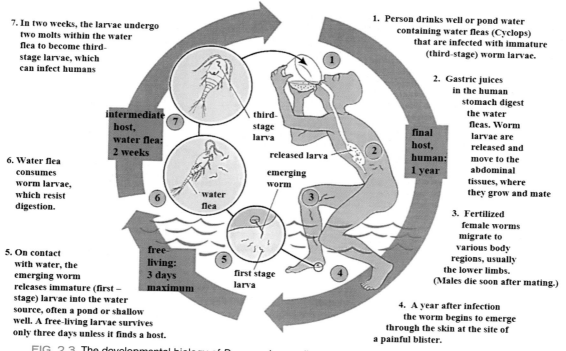

7. In two weeks, the larvae undergo two molts within the water flea to become third-stage larvae, which can infect humans

intermediate host, water flea: 2 weeks

6. Water flea consumes worm larvae, which resist digestion.

5. On contact with water, the emerging worm releases immature (first – stage) larvae into the water source, often a pond or shallow well. A free-living larvae survives only three days unless it finds a host.

free-living: 3 days maximum

first stage larva

water flea

emerging worm

released larva

third-stage larva

1. Person drinks well or pond water containing water fleas (Cyclops) that are infected with immature (third-stage) worm larvae.

2. Gastric juices in the human stomach digest the water fleas. Worm larvae are released and move to the abdominal tissues, where they grow and mate

final host, human: 1 year

3. Fertilized female worms migrate to various body regions, usually the lower limbs. (Males die soon after mating.)

4. A year after infection the worm begins to emerge through the skin at the site of a painful blister.

FIG. 2.3 The developmental biology of *Dracunculus medinensis*. (Source: Hopkins and Hopkins (1992).[4])

in Kaduna, Kogi, Kwara, and Niger States and in the Federal Capital Territory of Abuja. In those four States and in the Federal Capital Territory, as in the Southern States, free-flowing rivers and streams became stagnant pools and ponds during the dry season, thereby becoming a conducive ecological environment for breeding cyclops, contamination by infected persons and the transmission of GWD.

The peak seasonality of GWD has serious epidemiologic and socio-economic implications and consequences.

In those States where the peak transmission coincided with the rainy season, agriculture (the dominant local occupation) was adversely affected. The emergence of multiple and severe infections, with prolonged incapacitation, prevented farmers and their families (most of whom were also infected) from working on clearing the land, planting, weeding and even harvesting. Similarly, in States where the peak transmission occurred during the dry season, clearing land in preparation for planting and harvesting food and cash crops of significant economic value were

seriously affected with considerable loss of harvest, financial losses and wastage.

In 1987, the Rice Bowl Study sponsored by the United Nations Children's Fund (UNICEF Nigeria) estimated that in a small food basket in South Eastern Nigeria, farmers were losing US$20 million in profit on rice production alone every year.[1]

The knowledge of the magnitude, spread and seasonality of GWD is essential for promoting advocacy, raising awareness, planning interventions, mobilizing technical and material resources and attracting international support. Therefore, a reliable and an effective surveillance system must be used. Point prevalence should be interpreted cautiously because it may not be as reliable as an assessment based on monthly surveillance over a period of at least 1 year. Regular monitoring and supervision as well as program evaluation, should be an important component of the eradication drive against tropical diseases.

Sometimes, the constraints of poor accessibility or absolute inaccessibility due to bad weather, lack of roads, insecurity, insurgencies, natural disasters,

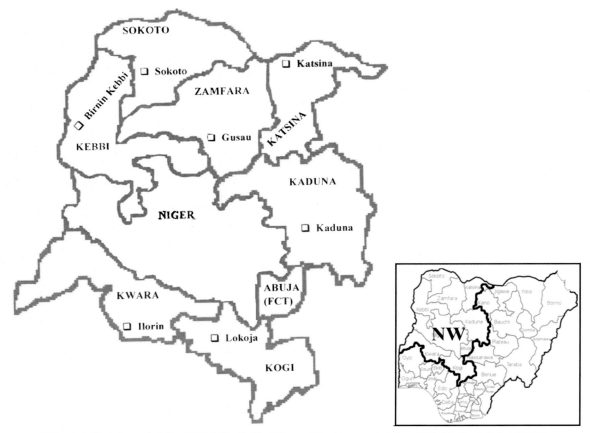

FIG. 2.4 Sketch map of the NIGEP North West Zone, Nigeria, showing the eight States and the Federal Capital Territory (FCT) in the zone at December 2000. Inset: Map of Nigeria showing the North West Zone and the State boundaries.

inadequate manpower and other barriers (Fig. 2.5A and B) could constitute a challenge and make all-year-round surveillance impossible.

The understanding of the biology of GWD transmission and of any tropical disease, is most valuable for identifying vulnerable links in the disease life cycle at which interventions can be targeted for control, elimination or eradication.

Based on our understanding of the biology of GWD transmission and in the absence of any effective vaccine or drug, multiple alternative strategies were used during the elimination drive in Nigeria. The strategies included: effective and continuous health education; safe water supply (use and maintenance); use of nylon monofilament filters (to sieve infected cyclops out of untreated drinking water) and vector control, using temephos (Abate) to kill the cyclops in the pond, thereby making the treated water source safe for consumption.

In addition, standardized monthly surveillance and other enhancing strategies (enumerated in the later chapters) are necessary.

Of all the core strategies adopted for the elimination of dracunculiasis, a safe water supply (use, adequacy, and maintenance) is the most permanent and most cost-effective strategy. This had been documented in the study of a UNICEF water project in Kwara State, Nigeria.[2] GWD is transmitted exclusively through drinking infested raw water. It is also the only disease that can be eliminated absolutely by providing and drinking safe water.

The adoption of all the core strategies used for the successful elimination of dracunculiasis in Nigeria required effective and continuous health

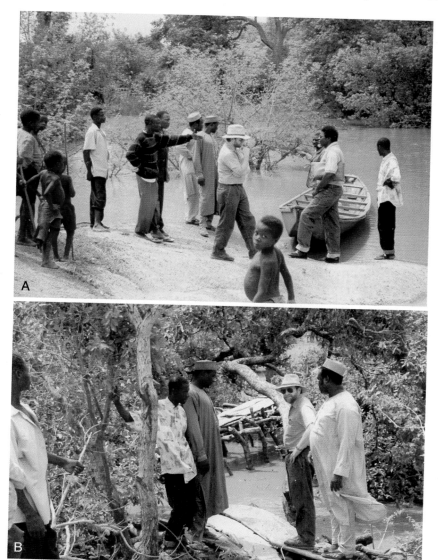

FIG. 2.5 **(A** and **B)**: Poor accessibility or outright inaccessibility to the endemic rural villages "at the end of the road" was a major challenge during the dracunculiasis elimination program. A severe outbreak had been reported in a village in Danko Wasagu Local Government Areas of Kebbi State. It coincided with the visit of Craig Withers, Jr. to the North West Zone. The team was scared of using the canoe to cross the river to the other side where the outbreak occurred.

education. This is an important lesson in the war against tropical diseases. The content of health education messages and the mode of their delivery are equally important.

Population movements by migrant farmers, nomadic Fulanis, long-distance drivers and traders, and cross-border regulations were serious challenges

encountered during dracunculiasis eradication. These should be carefully considered in the fight against other tropical diseases. Effective and sustained health education is a major intervention adopted to overcome the challenges of population movement.

Surgical extraction of Guinea worms, a radical innovative strategy, was used and became an important

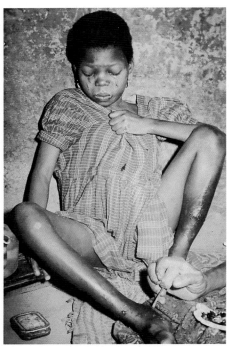

FIG. 2.6 Puncturing Guinea worm blisters with a red-hot iron (Sekia) is a common but dangerous traditional method of management; it invariably leads to serious pain, complications, and incapacitation.

3. It prevents protracted morbidity, complications and even death (from secondary bacterial infection);
4. It reduces the chances and rate of transmission significantly. Several Guinea worms were extracted and buried. Thus, there was no chance of L1 Guinea worm larvae getting into the ponds, contaminating the ponds or being transmitted;
5. The procedure was relatively cheap and at no cost to the victims and
6. Surgical extraction of Guinea worms was readily accepted and applauded by the State and Local Government Areas authorities, who used the efficacy of worm extraction to their political advantage.

In the war against other tropical diseases, alternative interventions that are cost-effective, safe and acceptable to the stakeholders should be kept in focus and explored.

REFERENCES

1. Edungbola LD, Braide EI, Nwosu AC, et al. *Guineaworm Control as a Major Contributor to Self-sufficiency in Rice Production in Nigeria*. New York: United Nations Children Fund; 1987. UNICEF/WATSAN/GW/2/87.
2. Edungbola LD, Watts SJ, Alabi TO, Bello AB. The impact of a UNICEF — assisted rural water project on the prevalence of Guinea worm disease in Asa, Kwara State, Nigeria. *Am J Trop Med Hyg.* 1988;39:79—85.
3. Ruiz-Tiben E, Hopkins DR. Dracunculiasis (Guinea Worm Disease) Eradication. *Advances in Parasitology.* 2006;61: 275—309.
4. Hopkins DR, Hopkins EM. *Guineaworm: The End in sight.* Chicago: Encyclopedia Britanica, Inc. Medical and Health Annual; 1992:10—27.
5. Muller R. In: *Advances in Parasitology.* vol. 9. London: Academic Press; 1971.

strategy in the rapid elimination of dracunculiasis, especially in the NIGEP North West Zone. Surgical extraction of Guinea worms has multiple advantages:
1. It is safe and far safer than the traditional methods (e.g., **Sekia**) that are used (Fig. 2.6);
2. It gives immediate relief (within 2—3 days);

CHAPTER 3

My Earliest Encounters With Dracunculiasis (Guinea Worm Disease)

FIRST ENCOUNTER

In 1954, my eldest brother was appointed (by a missionary of the Sudan Interior Mission) to start a religious class and a church in a small village (MG, now GM) in the Ifelodun Local Government Areas (LGA), Kwara State. Being an active young man with a rare passion for bicycles, my brother combined his primary assignments with bicycle repair in the village and surrounding communities where most successful farmers had bicycles. Bicycles were popular as part of marriage festivals when the bride would be carried on a heavily decorated bicycle and carried round the village up in the air, dancing for several hours. About a year later, my brother was brought to our village (about 20 km away) on a bicycle (no other vehicle or motorcycle in the area) with a badly swollen knee and a protruding threadlike worm, which was diagnosed locally as Sobiya (i.e., Guinea worm). Out of frustration and in intense pain, my brother pulled the worm by force as if to draw it out. The fragile worm was cut in two and one part withdrew into his tissue. The swelling and pain became so intense and unbearable that he was incapacitated and could not work for more than 3 months.

SECOND ENCOUNTER

In 1957, when I was in Primary Four (Standard Three), a friend and classmate from a village (now in Moro LGA of Kwara State) could not return to school after the first term holidays. He had multiple Guinea worm infections (his own village was endemic for Guinea worm disease [GWD]). He suffered adversely from ensuing secondary bacterial complications for months. He never returned to school and that was the end of his education.

THIRD ENCOUNTER

In 1960, the year Nigeria gained independence, I was in Senior Primary Seven. There was a crucial inter-school football match between two rival schools to celebrate independence locally. I played right-out while my friend played center forward. About 5 days before the crucial football match, two Guinea worms emerged on my friend's right foot and another on his left ankle. Our goalkeeper from my friend's village was also incapacitated. Both were from the same village endemic for Guinea worm. Sadly, they could not play! We were demoralized by their incapacitation and we lost the match, but the three of us got our First School Leaving Certificates that year.

FOURTH ENCOUNTER

Ironically, the same year, another classmate was to join me for an interview at the Provincial Secondary School Ilorin (now Government Secondary School Ilorin), having passed the government's written entrance examination. It was to be our first time ever to travel to Ilorin, the provincial headquarters.

About a week before traveling to Ilorin (a distance of about 120 km), on a very bad untarred road which was plied only by S.K. Dan Alhaji's lorry, my friend from a village endemic for Guinea worm could not travel. Thus, he lost a rare opportunity for a village boy to attend a Government Secondary School, virtually free of charge!

FIFTH ENCOUNTER

In 1970, my first cousin, a Primary School Grade 2 teacher, was transferred to a village notoriously endemic for dracunculiasis. Fear gripped him and the entire family. Out of unreserved determination to reject the posting (because of GWD), he boasted he would do everything humanly possible to make his transfer null and void. He did!

SIXTH ENCOUNTER

In 1976, while pursuing my Ph.D. at the Johns Hopkins School of Hygiene and Public Health, Baltimore, Maryland, USA, I wrote a Term Paper on dracunculiasis for the Tropical Medicine Course. The Professor in charge, Dr. Simpson, was so impressed that he awarded me the only A-grade in the course.

The Eradication of Dracunculiasis (Guinea Worm Disease) in Nigeria. https://doi.org/10.1016/B978-0-12-816764-9.00003-1

11

SEVENTH ENCOUNTER

In August 1978, I returned to Nigeria after successful completion of my Ph.D. in Pathobiology (Medical and Public Health Parasitology major).

At that time, there were no mobile phones and the telegram I sent to my family to pick me up at the airport was received 2 weeks after my arrival! Because I was not met at Murtala Mohammed Airport in Lagos, I took public transport going to Ilorin, a distance of about 400 km. About 70 km from Ilorin, our vehicle stopped at a village (Igbon) for passengers to relax. Curiously, I observed a Guinea worm dangling from the left hand of a woman who was selling pawpaw (papaya). The worm was partially covered by an old newspaper (Fig. 3.1).

Although I knew it was Guinea worm, I asked her what it was. Her response was snappy, "don't trouble me, everyone has it here." I politely asked if I could see 2 or 3 persons with it. Almost immediately, some five persons, including a 3 year old girl (Fig. 3.2A and B) were presented.

With mixed feelings of personal excitement and concern for the victims, I returned to the village with my elder brother, a principal nurse at the General Hospital Ilorin, who performed case management in form of washing wounds, cleaning and dressing, on many people with Guinea worm, while I identified the ponds where transmissions were occurring, gave health education, and discussed the possibility of a hand-dug well with the village head. He was not convinced and boasted of a village with "Omi Awoye" (water that

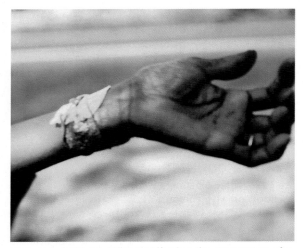

FIG. 3.1 Pawpaw seller manifesting the emergence of a Guinea worm on her hand and using old newspaper (as a treatment) to cover the ulcer and the emerging worm.

heals). About 3 weeks later, he had three emerging worms with bad ulcers on both legs. Community legislation was passed against entering and contaminating the two community ponds for a fine of a goat! Families were also advised to boil their drinking water. Two hand-dug wells were constructed and a borehole was later set up by the Oyo State Government. Dr. Susan Watts and Bola Adana joined me actively in promoting interventions. Within 3 years, 3 striking things happened in the community:

1. GWD transmission was interrupted in the community and permanently thereafter;
2. Late Governor Bola Ige (SAN) of Oyo State established a Government Day Secondary School in the community and
3. The experience was documented in two publications in the *Journal of Tropical Medicine and Hygiene*.[1,2]

EIGHTH ENCOUNTER

As a lecturer in Medical and Public Health Parasitology in the Faculty of Health Sciences, University of Ilorin, Ilorin, Nigeria, I took advantage of my previous encounters with dracunculiasis, the Community Based Experience and Services (a WHO Collaborating Center for Man-Power Development and Research) and my knowledge of several neighboring and remote communities endemic for Guinea worms to form a research team of interested academic colleagues. They included: Drs. Susan Watts; Bode Kayode; O. Agbede; W. Ebomoyi; D.B. Parakoyi; T. Alabi and K.S. Adeyemi. The goals of the team were to carry out prevalence surveys of dracunculiasis in the neighboring and remote villages in Kwara State, to ascertain the knowledge, attitudes and practices of the people about the disease, to establish the socioeconomic impact of the disease, to promote advocacy and awareness about the disease and to assess the prospects of introducing interventions to control the disease.

Having established the magnitude of the problem, a proposal for funding was written and sent to a high-profile international organization. Although the proposal was commended, funding it was declined because dracunculiasis was regarded as a local problem by the organization. However, the agency magnanimously advised that the proposal could be submitted to the National Institute of Medical Research in Lagos.

The Director of the Institute, a professor, received me warmly and commended the quality of the proposal but regretted that I did not know my "literature," angrily asking what I wanted to do that Professor Onabamiro had not already done. I replied politely that Professor Onabamiro had done some useful work on cyclops,

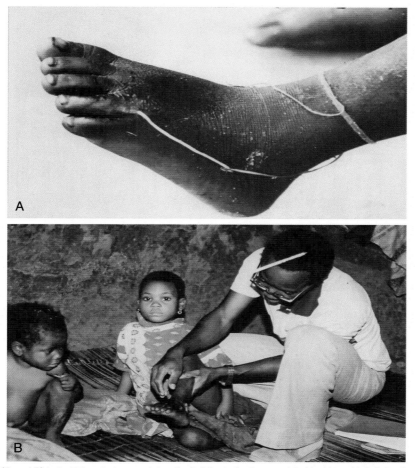

FIG. 3.2 **(A** and **B)** Luke Edungbola examining the left foot of a 3-year-old girl with multiple infections in 1978. Both feet were infected.

the intermediate host of *Dracunculus medinensis*, but my team wanted to embark on awareness promotion and on targeting the disease for control and, thereby, alleviate the year after year agony of human suffering and impoverishment caused by GWD. The last words from the Director were "good luck, young man. We have no funding for projects that are neither feasible nor promising."

Undaunted by the rejection, our epidemiological studies went on, using personal resources. On one occasion, Mr. Richard S. Reid (UNICEF Country Representative) and three of his staff were visiting my office for the first time. Coincidentally, we were just returning from fieldwork in heavy rainfall in my lift-back sports car brought back from the United States in 1978. The car was muddy and dirty. Mr. Reid was

touched by our efforts and transport constraints. He told me to go and collect a brand new Land Cruiser in Lagos for our fieldwork. That was a great motivation and encouragement that strengthened our modest efforts.

In the course of our community surveys for dracunculiasis, an alarming outbreak was encountered at Kankan, a village in Asa LGA, about 20 km away. To bring this terrible outbreak to the public attention, I invited a journalist from the *Sunday Concord* (the most popular Sunday newspaper) to cover the outbreak. He did with a sensational front page headline in color "Kankan, the City of Guinea Worm in Kwara" (Fig. 3.3). The publication was brought to the attention of the then Military Governor of Kwara State, Group Captain Salaudeen Adebola Latinwo. When the

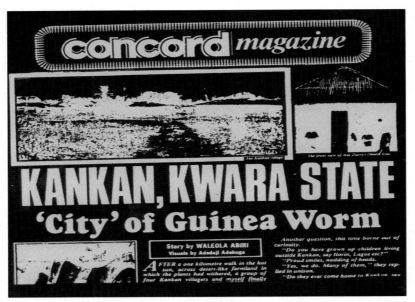

FIG. 3.3 A sensational article in the leading Sunday Newspaper in Nigeria which stimulated national awareness and political response to the problem of Guinea worm disease at a magnitude unprecedented in the country.

Governor was made aware that I knew about the publication, he invited me to Government House that Sunday. He was furious that I was embarrassing the State but I insisted that the story was real. We drove in his vehicle to the village. When he came face to face with the reality, he shed tears. Unfortunately, he had no handkerchief in his pocket but I gave him some tissue papers from my camera bag.

That publication and the Governor's visit accelerated the commencement of UNICEF/WATSAN (Water, Sanitation, and Hygiene) program in Kwara State. That and the ensuing political commitment to the dracunculiasis problem resulted in Kwara State having one of the most committed and aggressive interventions for accelerated elimination of the disease in Nigeria.

My intimate and strong earliest encounters with dracunculiasis and its horrors at the grass roots level, the encouragement of UNICEF at the onset and the consistent technical, material and financial support of The Carter Center throughout the successful eradication campaign, were the impetus that motivated and sustained my commitment to dracunculiasis elimination until Nigeria was certified free of the disease by the WHO in 2013.

REFERENCES

1. Edungbola LD. Dracunculiasis in Igbon, Oyo state, Nigeria. *J Trop Med Hyg.* 1984;87:153−158.
2. Edungbola LD, Watts SJ. The elimination of dracunculiasis in Igbon, Oyo State, Nigeria: the success of self-help activities. *J Trop Med Hyg.* 1990;93:1−6.

CHAPTER 4

History of Dracunculiasis (Guinea Worm Disease) and Notable International Records

HISTORY OF DRACUNCULIASIS

Guinea worm and Guinea worm disease (GWD; dracunculiasis) have an exceptional, fascinating, and extensive history documented by a wide range of professionals and personalities in virtually in all continents of the world where the disease occurred. Among the various groups that have contributed to the rich history of the Guinea worm and GWD are explorers, navigators, voyagers, tourists, travelers, physicians, parasitologists, historians, epidemiologists, botanists, anthropologists, sociologists, geographers, archaeologists, museum curators, archivists, librarians, religion personnel, military officers, slave traders, mathematicians, demographers, public health practitioners, economists, administrators, etc.

The wide-ranging attraction and interest in Guinea worms and GWD are attributable to multiple factors, including:

1. the ancient past of dracunculiasis;
2. the peculiarities of its endemicity and geographic spread in Africa, Asia, Europe and the Americas, at one time or the other (in ancient times, recently or currently);
3. the historical significance of dracunculiasis in religions and in the sciences, including medicine and public health;
4. the impact of the disease on health, education, agriculture, socioeconomic activities and general development;
5. the association of the disease with ignorance, apathy, poverty, insecurity and abject neglect;
6. the propensity of the infection for transmission, dissemination, multiple infections and emergence at virtually all anatomic locations on the human body;
7. the parasitic phenomenality of *Dracunculiasis medinensis* which terrorized man for decades, despite its vulnerability to effective interventions and political commitment;
8. high annual incidence of the infection year after year. Stoll[1] estimated that there were 43.3 million cases in the world. Ralph Muller[2] contended that the number of cases estimated by Stoll[1] was not reducing;
9. dracunculiasis is one of the easiest infectious diseases to diagnose, even by the villagers;
10. the World Health Organization (WHO) targeted dracunculiasis for eradication and made it a subgoal of the Water Decade in 1986 and
11. dracunculiasis is (potentially) only the second infectious disease, after smallpox,[3] and the first parasitic helminthiasis to be eradicated.

According to Hopkins and Hopkins,[3] Ebers Papyrus "one of the oldest known collections of medical texts, at about 1550 BC, in ancient Egypt," provided the earliest evidence of dracunculiasis. The collection describes the proper procedure of extracting a Guinea worm by winding it around a stick. This practice remained universal in rural parts of Nigeria, Africa, and other parts of the world until recently.

It is historically instructive, striking and significant that Guinea worm epitomizes the symbol of medicine, i.e. the staff of Asclepius (the Greco-Roman God of medicine (Fig. 4.1) as well as the logo (Fig. 4.2) adopted by the WHO to epitomize its unequivocal commitment to the highest level of health care and delivery globally.[3]

5 And the people spoke against God, and against Moses: "Why have you brought us up out of Egypt to die in the wilderness? For there is no food and water, and our soul loathes this worthless bread."

6 So the Lord sent fiery serpents among the people, and they bit the people; and much people of Israel died.

7 Therefore the people came to Moses, and said, "We have sinned, for we have spoken against the Lord, and against you; pray unto the Lord, that He take away the serpents from us." So Moses prayed for the people.

The Eradication of Dracunculiasis (Guinea Worm Disease) in Nigeria. https://doi.org/10.1016/B978-0-12-816764-9.00004-3

8 Then the Lord said unto Moses, "Make a fiery serpent, and set it on a pole; and it shall be that everyone who is bitten, when he looks upon it, shall live."

9 So Moses made a bronze serpent, and put it on a pole, and so it was, if a serpent had bitten anyone, when he looked at the bronze serpent, he lived.

(THE HOLY BIBLE, NUMBERS 21:5−9).

The above account from the 12th or 13th century was the seventh iniquity of ingratitude, grumbling and complaining against God and His servant, Moses, by the Israelites since their mass exodus from slavery in Egypt *En route* to Canaan, the promised land full of milk and honey.

The journey, miraculously through the Red Sea and encampments on the shore of the Red Sea, lasted for 40 years of wandering in the wilderness (because of their sins) instead of 40 days.

The aforementioned "fiery serpent" which God sent to bite and kill many Israelites during the above episode, has been interpreted by a number of authorities as a Guinea worm. Dracunculiasis was known to be endemic in the Middle East, especially along the shores of the Red Sea where the Canaan-bound Israelites encamped for 40 years. Apparently, dracunculiasis existed before the exodus of the Israelites from Egypt.

Avicenna (980−1037), in his *Canon of Medicine* reported that dracunculiasis occurred in Egypt and even said that "should the worm be ruptured, much pain and trouble ensue, and even if rupture does not take place, the condition is tiresome enough."[3]

Strong persuasive evidence that the biblical "fiery serpent" was indeed a Guinea worm was presented by Alfred J. Bollett, a Professor of clinical medicine at Yale University School of Medicine.[3]

Plutarch (AD 50−117), Galen (AD 129−199), and other Greco-Roman writers mentioned dracunculiasis. Avincenna (980−1037) gave the first detailed clinical presentations of "Medina sickness" (*Vena Medina*), so-called because it was highly prevalent in Medina from where it was believed to have been disseminated to other parts of the world through pilgrimage routes.[4]

In 1674, G.H. Velschius, from Vienna, published *Exercitaito de Vena Medinensis*, a comprehensive account of dracunculiasis with an illustration showing Persian physicians extracting a Guinea worm (Fig. 4.3) by winding it around specially designed instruments.

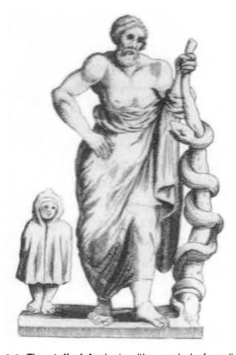

FIG. 4.1 The staff of Asclepius (the symbol of medicine). National Library of Medicine, Bethesda, Maryland, USA. (From: Hopkins DR, Hopkins EM. *Guineaworm: The End in Sight*. Chicago: Encyclopedia Britannica, Inc. Medical and Health Annual; 1992:10−27.)

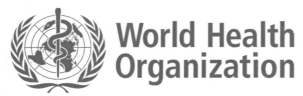

FIG. 4.2 World Health Organization logo.

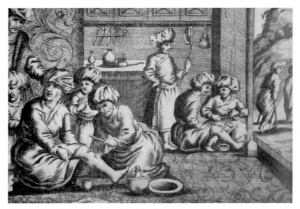

FIG. 4.3 Persian physician extracting a Guinea worm (from Velschius 1647). (From: Muller R. *Advances in Parasitology*, Vol. 9. London: Academic Press, 1971.)

In 1870, Fedshenko (a Russian) associated *Cyclops* with the life cycle of the Guinea worm. Historically, that was the first time an invertebrate host was implicated in the transmission of a medically important disease.[5]

In 1611, a European traveler from Switzerland was the first to call the disease "Guinea worm" when he observed dracunculiasis among West Africans, along the Gulf of Guinea, which currently encompasses 16 West African countries that constitute the Economic Community of West African States (ECOWAS) by the Lagos Treaty of 1975.

Guinea is a geographic expression in West Africa with characteristic vegetation, climate, people, animals, and crops.

Historically, a guinea is an obsolete English gold coin, first made of gold from Guinea, in West Africa. Its last value was 21 shillings.

"Guinea" is not exclusive to the Guinea worm as a prefix. Other names prefixed by "Guinea" include:

Guinea corn (sorghum, a cereal);

Guinea fowl (a beautiful African bird);

Guinea savannah (vegetation of tall grasses and scattered woods dominated by locust bean and shea butter trees);

Guinea pig (a small South American rodent);

Guinea grass (a tall African grass of millet genus *Penicum*);

Guinea brocade (a popular type of cloth material in West Africa);

Guinea (a West African country with Conakry as the capital) and

Guinea Bissau (a West African country with Bissau as the capital).

A Scottish explorer and surgeon, Dr. Mungo Park (1771−1806), mentioned Guinea worms in the documentation of his two travels (1795 and 1803) in interior West Africa to unravel the source of River Niger. He died tragically at the age of 35 years when his boat hit a rock and capsized on the River Niger rapids at Bussa as he was simultaneously being attacked with bows, arrows, and spears by hostile villagers.

Mungo Park was buried on the banks of the River Niger in Jebba (Kwara State). Monuments to him are found today in New Bussa, Jebba, Lokoja, etc.

One of the earliest epidemiological records of dracunculiasis in Nigeria was that of Ramsay.[6] However, the disease, its horrors, ecology and impact had been recognized much earlier. National archives in Kaduna (Northern Nigeria), during colonial rule, contain fascinating reports, including NAK Ilorin Province 5.211.5A (Ilorin Emirate Notes, 1937),[7] and the Guinea worm file PCJ no. 174[8] had earlier documented the ecology and impact of dracunculiasis and recommended control measures. One of the control measures was the destruction of cyclops, using the fruits of a local tree (aduwa). The ancient records also contain a report of the emergence of Guinea worms on some prisoners from Ilorin Province who were serving their jail terms in the Regional Headquarters' Prison (epidemiology of Guinea worm in Ilorin Emirate).

The archives also documented the problem of dracunculiasis in Ngaski (now in Kebbi State) when a colonial administrator directed that "boiling water should be poured into the wells." It has been argued that the directive could have been a misinterpretation of what should correctly be to boil water before consumption.

Until it was recently eliminated by the Nigeria Guinea Worm Eradication Programme, with the assistance of The Carter Center and other agencies, dracunculiasis remained rampant in the Ngaski, Yauri, and Birni Yauri districts of Kebbi State (formerly part of Sokoto State).

Whereas dracunculiasis had a long-standing history in many parts of Nigeria, one of the earliest concerted local endeavors was the research work of Professor S.D. Onabamiro, a zoologist, at the Nigeria Premier University of Ibadan where he carried out his investigations (in the 1950s) on the identification of various species of *Cyclops* (including the ones scientifically named after him and the community) in the transmission of Guinea worm by *Thermocyclops nigerianas* and on the geographic distribution of dracunculiasis in the South Western Region of Nigeria. Since the 1980s, a wealth of rich information has been published on the epidemiology, transmission, impact and intervention measures targeted at eliminating the disease nation-wide.

NOTABLE INTERNATIONAL RECORDS ON DRACUNCULIASIS

1926: USSR launched a campaign to eliminate dracunculiasis with about 10,000 cases in Bukhara and using multiple interventions, including health education and safe water supply. By 1933, the disease was successfully eliminated in the Soviet Union.

1977: United Nations Water Conference in Mardel Plata, Argentina, proclaimed 1981–99 as the International Drinking Water Supply and Sanitation Decade with the goal of safe drinking water and sanitation for all by the year 1990.

1980: World Health Organization inaugurated the International Drinking Supply and Sanitation Decade.

1981: The Steering Committee for the Water and Sanitation Decade adopted dracunculiasis eradication as a sub-goal.

1984: Professor Edungbola was nominated by Dr. Donald R. Hopkins at the Centers for Disease Control and Prevention (CDC) to present a paper on dracunculiasis and the challenges of its eradication at the Impact Conference in Nairobi, Kenya.

1985: First National Conference on Dracunculiasis in Africa was held in Ilorin, Kwara State, Nigeria.

1986: The 39th World Health Assembly adopted a resolution formally targeting dracunculiasis as a major infectious disease second only to smallpox to be eradicated.

1986: The First African Regional Conference on Dracunculiasis Eradication was held in Niamey, Niger Republic. Six participants attended from Nigeria.

1987: Pakistan launched a dracunculiasis eradication program.

1987: The International Symposium on Water and Sanitation in Africa was held in Atlanta, Georgia, USA. The symposium provided a forum for a mid-decade assessment of Water Supply and Sanitation activities in Africa and also featured several papers on dracunculiasis.

1988: African Ministers of Health, under the auspices of the WHO, adopted a resolution to eradicate dracunculiasis in Africa by 1995. Professor Olikoye Ransome-Kuti, Hon. Minister of Health (Nigeria), co-sponsored the resolution.

1988: India conducted its Third Independent Appraisal of the Status of Dracunculiasis Eradication. Professor Luke Edungbola was sponsored by CDC/Global 2000 to participate.

1988: The Second African Regional Conference on dracunculiasis was held in Accra, Ghana. The president of the host country, Flight Lieutenant Jerry Rawlings, the 39th President of the United States of America, Hon. Jimmy Carter and his wife (Rosalyn Carter), Professor G.L. Monekosso and Dr. Donald R. Hopkins attended the conference. During the conference, a universal definition of a case of dracunculiasis (an individual exhibiting or having a recent, i.e., within a year, history of skin lesion with emergence of Guinea worm), was adopted. The conference sponsors were WHO, United States Agency for International Aid, Global 2000, CDC (Atlanta), UNICEF (Nigeria), and Peace Corps (Benin).

1988: President Jimmy Carter (Representing Global 2000/The Carter Center) signed a Memorandum of understanding with the Federal Government of Nigeria, represented by Professor Olikoye Ransome-Kuti (the erstwhile Hon. Minister of Health), for a partnership in a dracunculiasis eradication program in Nigeria by 1995.

1989: International Donors' Conference was held in Lagos Sheraton. A sum of US$10 million was raised for dracunculiasis eradication. The Federal Government of Nigeria, The Carter Center (led by President Jimmy Carter and his wife), UNICEF and the United Nations Development Programme (UNDP) co-sponsored the conference. The UNDP Regional Director, Pierra-Claver Dambia, chaired the conference.

1990: American Cyanamid Co., the world's only manufacturer of temaphos (Abate) donated, through The Carter Center, enough larvicide to eradicate dracunculiasis in all affected African countries up to 1995. UNICEF was to assist in shipping the donated temephos to endemic African countries.

1990: In partnership with the Precision Fabrics Group, E.I. DuPont de Nemours & Co donated a million nylon filters and also pledged to supply millions more filters for water filtration throughout the dracunculiasis eradication drive.

1990: The WHO established criteria for assessing and certifying previously, recently and currently endemic countries free of dracunculiasis after at least 3 years of consecutive zero case reporting.

1991:
- The Fourth National Guinea Worm Conference (Second National Guinea Worm Day) was observed at the Institute of International Affairs, Lagos.
- The Federal Government of Nigeria demonstrated its commitment to dracunculiasis elimination in the country by launching three commemorative postage stamps on March 20, 1991.
- The Vice President directed that all 589 LGAs in the 30 States and the Federal Capital Territory should mandatorily devote 10% of their health budget to dracunculiasis eradication.

1991: The 44th World Health Assembly adopted a resolution for the eradication of dracunculiasis country by country and fixed the goal of interrupting transmission by 1995.

1991: A review of Ghanaian and Nigerian Guinea Worm Eradication Programs at The Carter Center, Atlanta, Georgia, USA, under the chairmanship of President Jimmy Carter and his wife, Rosalynn Carter (Fig. 4.4).

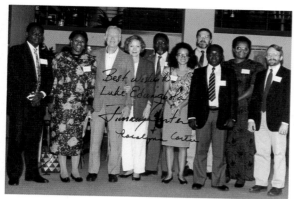

FIG. 4.4 President Jimmy Carter (chairman, The Carter Center) and his wife, Rosalynn Carter, with The NIGEP zonal facilitators and two Global 2000/The Carter Center technical advisors (Craig Withers Jr. and Pat McConnon) during the 1991 Ghana—Nigeria Programme Review in Atlanta.

1995: WHO established an independent International Commission for the Certification of Dracunculiasis Eradication (ICCDE). The Commission also has the mandate of recommending those countries that have fulfilled their certification requirements.

1996: WHO created a panel of specialists from which members could be assigned to the International Certification Teams.

2002: Seventh Dracunculiasis Eradication Programme Managers' Meeting was held in Khartoum, Sudan.

2011: Nigeria and some African countries received The Carter Center Award for dracunculiasis eradication after reporting no indigenous cases of the disease for more than two consecutive years. The award was made at The Carter Center, Atlanta, Georgia, USA, during the 15th Meeting of Programme Managers of Dracunculiasis Eradication.

2013: WHO declared Nigeria free of dracunculiasis, based on the recommendation of the WHO International Certification Commission.

REFERENCES

1. Stoll NR. This wormy world. *J Parasitol.* 1947;32:1—18.
2. Muller R. In: *Advances in Parasitology.* vol. 9. London: Academic Press; 1971.
3. Hopkins DR, Hopkins EM. *Guineaworm: The End in Sight..* Chicago: Encyclopedia Britannica, Inc. Medical and Health Annual; 1992:10—27.
4. Hopkins DR. Dracunculiasis: an eradication scourge. *Epidemiol Rev.* 1983;5:208—219.
5. Litvinor SK, Lysenko AY. Dracunculiasis I. History of the discovery of the intermediate host and the eradication of foci of invasion in the USSR. In: *Paper Prepared for Presentation at the Workshop on the Opportunities for the Control of Dracunculiasis, National Research Council, Washington DC, June 16—19. 1982.*
6. Ramsay GWSC. Observations on an intradermal test for dracontiasis. *Trans R Soc Trop Med Hyg.* 1935;28:399—404.
7. National Archives Kaduna: NAK Ilorin Province 5.211.5A (Ilorin Emirate Notes). 1937.
8. National Archives Kaduna: The Guineawprm File. PCJ No. 174.

CHAPTER 5

Global Occurrence of Dracunculiasis

- Ancient, recent and current documentations have shown that endemic dracunculiasis occurred in most of the continents of the world, namely, Africa, Asia, Europe and North and South America. Although dracunculiasis had been known elsewhere much earlier, it is suggested that the disease was "introduced into several countries of the mainland, North, Central and South Americas during African slave trade."[1]
- Between early 1900s and 2016, endemic dracunculiasis was confined exclusively to Africa and Asia (Fig. 5.1).
- Of the 129,903 cases of dracunculiasis reported to the World Health Organization (WHO) in 1996, 99.9% occurred in Africa, of which about three-quarters were in South Sudan.[1]
- Interventions in South Sudan were hampered by the war in that part of Africa. It eventually took the intervention of President Jimmy Carter and the Organization of Africa Unity to broker a cease fire during which effective interventions were implemented.
- The provision, utilization and maintenance of safe water supplies and sustained improvement in the standard of living, led to the elimination of endemic dracunculiasis in Europe and the Americas.
- In 1995, an independent International Commission for the Certification of Dracunculiasis Eradication (ICCDE) was established by the WHO.[2]
- At its first meeting in 1996 in Geneva, the Commission revised the criteria for certification. A panel of specialists from which members could be assigned to International Certification Teams (ICTs) was also constituted.
- As shown in Fig. 5.1 D, globally, as at 2016, dracunculiasis endemic in only four African countries (Chad, Ethiopia, Mali and South Sudan). Kenya and North Sudan are in the pre-certification stage and Angola and the Democratic Republic of the Congo (both never known to be endemic), are pending dracunculiasis-free certification.[3]

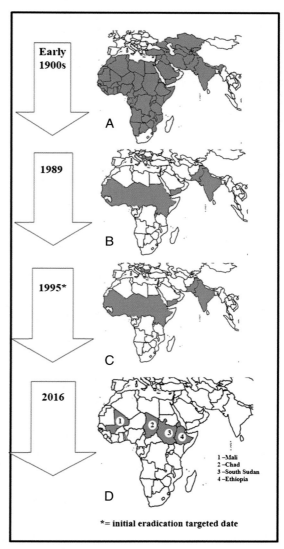

FIG. 5.1 Global trends of dracunculiasis endemicity (1900–2016).

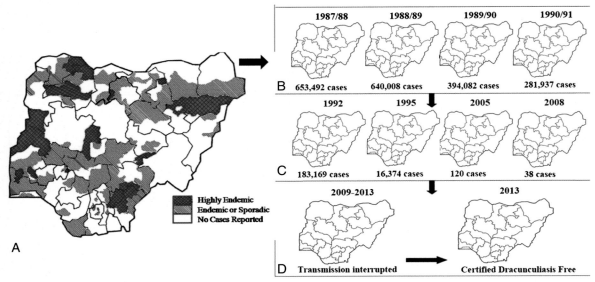

FIG. 5.2 Trends of dracunculiasis endemicity and elimination in Nigeria between 1985 and 2013. (A) Endemicity of GWD in Nigeria, based on the 1985 National GWD Conference Report. (B) Endemicity of GWD in Nigeria, based on Active Case Searches of 1987/88–1990/91 and showing steady decline in the number of cases. (C) Endemicity of GWD in Nigeria (1992-2008), based on Active Monthly Surveillance and showing dramatic decline in the number of cases. (D) Interruption of GWD transmission in Nigeria (2009-2013) and the Certification of Nigeria Free of GWD in 2013.

TABLE 5.1
Dracunculiasis-Free Certification by Geographic Areas (1997–2013)

S. No.	Geographic Areas	No. (%) of Countries Certified Free
1	Africa	40 (21.5)
2	Americas	35 (18.8)
3	Europe	52 (28.0)
4	Eastern Mediterranean	21 (11.3)
5	Western Pacific	27 (14.5)
6	South East Asia	11 (5.9)
Total		186 (100)

- In 2013, Nigeria was certified free of dracunculiasis by the ICCDE.

The global status of dracunculiasis-free certification by the WHO is shown in Table 5.1. Of the 186 countries certified free of dracunculiasis globally, 15 (8.1%) were previously endemic.[3]

REFERENCES

1. World Health Organization. *Certification of Dracunculiasis Eradication: Criteria, Strategies, Procedures.* WHO/FIL/96/188; 1996.
2. World Health Organization. *Criteria for the Certification of Dracunculiasis Eradication.* WHO/FIL/96/187 Rev. 1; 1996.
3. World Health Organization. *Dracunculiasis Eradication.* who.int/dracunculiasis/certification/en; 2018.

- The trends of dracunculiasis endemicity and elimination in Nigeria, between 1985 and 2013, are depicted in Fig. 5.2

CHAPTER 6

Dracunculiasis in Nigeria: A Calendar of Some Major National Events

1934: Ramsay, the Director of Medical and Sanitation Services, confirmed the prevalence and endemicity of dracunculiasis in Ilorin Province, especially in the Ilorin Emirate, where affected districts and prevention measures were reported (National Archive Kaduna, IlorProf 174A, Guinea worm in Nigeria).

1950s: Professor S.D. Onabamiro, a zoologist at the University of Ibadan, studied various species of *Cyclops*, especially *Thermocylcops nigerianus* in relation to the transmission of dracunculiasis. He also reported the geographic distribution of the disease in south western Nigeria.

1984: UNICEF (Nigeria)'s Country Representative (Mr. Richard S. Reid) at a UNICEF Workshop in Ikoyi Hotel, Lagos, agreed to using dracunculiasis as a more potent indicator of the efficacy of safe water supply and sanitation than diarrhea. Also, it was accepted that the elimination of dracunculiasis would serve as an attractive "entry point" for endemic communities to participate more actively in Primary Health Care (PHC) activities, especially the Expanded Programme on Immunization (EPI) at that time.

1984: An International Workshop on the Development of Research on Human Science Applied to PHC was held at the University of Maiduguri under the Vice-Chancellorship of Professor Jubril Aminu (former Nigerian Ambassador to the United Nations). UNICEF, WHO, and the Federal Government of Nigeria sponsored the workshop.

After Professor Edungbola's invited presentation on water-related health problems in PHC, with emphasis on dracunculiasis, his recommendation for a national conference on dracunculiasis was approved in principle. Professor J.D. Adeniyi, Professor Egunjobi and Dr. D.A. Kolawole were asked to work with Professor Edungbola to prepare a detailed proposal with program of events, time, participants and budget. The proposal was to be submitted to Mr. David Bassiouni (Senior Program Officer, UNICEF) for the attention of Mr. Richard Reid (the Country Representative).

1984: Dr. D.R. Hopkins and Professor L.D. Edungbola met for the first time (in the WHO office of Professor Umaru Shehu, the Country Coordinator), exchanged Guinea worm photographs and shared a mutual commitment to dracunculiasis eradication.

1984: Professors Kale and Edungbola designed postal survey questionnaires on dracunculiasis endemicity in Nigeria and distributed the questionnaires through the WHO office in Lagos, Nigeria, with the assistance of Professor Umaru Sehu (the WHO coordinator).

1984: "Kankan, the City of Guinea worm in Nigeria," a sensational article on dracunculiasis, was published as the front page headline in the Sunday Concord (the most widely read Sunday daily in Nigeria) on June 10, 1984. The publication spurred the Kwara State Government and UNICEF (Nigeria) to take a lead in dracunculiasis eradication, using aggressive political commitment, health education and safe water supply. This positive outcome attested to the role and power of the press.

1985: UNICEF (Nigeria) donated a Toyota Land Cruiser to the University of Ilorin dracunculiasis research team in appreciation and as encouragement to the team's commitment to the mapping of dracunculiasis endemicity and its eradication drive in the State.

1985: The First National Conference on Dracunculiasis in Nigeria (the first of its kind in Africa) was held in Ilorin, Kwara State. The Military Governor of Kwara State (Group Captain Salaudeen Adebola Latinwo), the Hon. Minister of Health (Dr. Emmanuel Nsan, represented by Dr. A.D. Kolawole), the Vice Chancellor, University of Ilorin (Professor S. Afolabi Toye), UNICEF Country Representative (Mr. Richard Reid), Deputy Director, Centers for Disease Control and Prevention (CDC), Atlanta, GA, USA (Dr. Donald R. Hopkins) Dr. Donald Belcher (University of California, USA) and Dr. R.N. Basu (Director, National Institute of Communicable Diseases, Delhi, India), attended the

The Eradication of Dracunculiasis (Guinea Worm Disease) in Nigeria. https://doi.org/10.1016/B978-0-12-816764-9.00006-7

23

3-day conference. Participants were drawn from all the States and the Federal Capital Territory (FCT); Local Government Areas (LGAs); Ministries; Research Institutes; Universities and the Offices of UNICEF, WHO and CDC. UNICEF; WHO; Federal Ministry of Health and the University of Ilorin sponsored the conference in collaboration with the CDC.

A significant outcome of the conference was the unequivocal revelation that dracunculiasis was endemic in virtually all States and FCT in Nigeria. The country's endemicity map of dracunculiasis produced at the conference gave details far exceeding what had ever been known previously.

1986: The First African Regional Conference on Dracunculiasis was held in Niamey, Niger Republic. Six Nigerians (Professors A.B.C. Nwosu, Kale, Adeniyi and Edungbola, Dr. Timi Agary and Mr. Osin) attended.

During their return journey and their unjustifiable delay for 3 days in Abidjan by the country's immigration officers at the airport (until the Nigerian Embassy in Cote de Voire came to their rescue), Professor Kale and Edungbola utilized the delay to develop the involvement of the National Youth Service Corps (NYSC) in dracunculiasis eradication and discussed the potential of using Nigerian commemorative postage stamps to promote advocacy and public enlightenment.

1986: The first State Taskforce on dracunculiasis eradication in Nigeria was inaugurated in Anambra State through the influence of Professor A.B.C. Nwosu, a Parasitologist, and the State's Hon. Commissioner for Health who launched aggressive interventions using health education, safe water supply and vector control with temephos (Abate).

1986: Professor Olikoye Ransome-Kuti became the Hon. Minister of Health and declared unprecedented support and commitment to the implementation of PHC activities, dracunculiasis eradication, and onchocerciasis control, among other remarkable programs he pioneered in Nigeria.

1986: Facilitated by Dr. S.H. Brew-Graves (WHO representative in Nigeria) and Dr. K.A. Ojodu, the new Minister of Health, Professor Edungbola was invited to give an update on the status of dracunculiasis and onchocerciasis in Nigeria. The presentation took place in the Minister's Conference Room on the 10th floor at the Federal Secretariat, Ikoyi, Lagos. The interaction strengthened the commitment to launching dracunculiasis eradication and onchocerciasis control programs in Nigeria.

1987: Professor L.D. Edungbola spent a 1-year sabbatical with Global 2000, working with Joe Giordano (Director of Operations) and Dr. Donald R. Hopkins (Senior Consultant, Global 2000) to develop the Nigeria dracunculiasis eradication program.

1987: Professor L.D. Edungbola presented luncheon seminars on dracunculiasis and onchocerciasis at Vector Biology & Control (under USAID), Arlington, Virginia, USA. The seminar helped to eliminate prejudices and reservations among some influential groups against the feasibility of eradicating dracunculiasis. With sound scientific evidence presented, Drs. Brian Duke and Alfred Buck agreed that Guinea worm disease is eradicable. Bob Lennox, Victor Baberio, Barry Silverman, and Dr. Arata also affirmed their strong belief that dracunculiasis can be eradicated.

1987: The Rice Bowl Study, sponsored by UNICEF and conducted by Dr. L.D. Edungbola, Dr. Braide, Dr. K.S. Adeyemi, Dr. A.C. Nwosu (of Nigeria Institute of Socio-Economic Research, NISER) Dr. E.I.I. Gemade and Carel de Rooy (Chief of Water & Sanitation, UNICEF, Nigeria).

The study estimated that due to dracunculiasis morbidity (in a small "food basket" of South East Nigeria), farmers were losing US\$20m in profit on rice production alone every year. Other crops such as maize, yam, cassava, beans and major economic trees, were similarly adversely affected.

1988: The maiden meeting of the National Task Force on Dracunculiasis Eradication in Nigeria was held on May 5 and 6, 1988, in the Board Room of the Federal Epidemiological Unit, Onikan Health Center, Lagos.

The participants were: Dr. A.D. Kolawole (Chief Consultant, Epidemiological Unit); Professor L.D. Edungbola; Dr. Eka Braide; Dr. C.N. Obionu (Anambra State Director of Health Services); Dr. M.K.O. Padonu; Dr. Lola Sadiq; Dr. O. Ogunnowo; Dr. B.B. Bhalerao (WHO) and L. Donaldson (UNICEF, Nigeria).

In attendance were: Dr. (Mrs.) O.O. Ojo; Dr. Y. Saka and Miss. E.P. Otok-Akpan. Professor O. Kale and Dr. Timi Agary (Federal Ministry of Science and Technology) were absent with apology. Dr. Don. R. Hopkins (Senior Consultant, Global 2000) and Craig Withers, Jr. (the first Resident Technical Advisor for Global 2000) attended the second meeting on July 1, 1988.

The Nigeria Guinea Worm Eradication Programme (NIGEP) was adopted as the national body in the Federal Ministry of Health to coordinate the activities of the Nigerian dracunculiasis eradication program.

The composition of the enlarged National Task Force will be multi-sectoral and to include representatives of the 22 states (including the FCT, Abuja); Federal Ministries of Health, Agriculture, Water Resources, Education, Science & Technology; Universities and Research Institutes; United Nations (UNICEF, WHO, and United Nations Development Programme

[UNDP]); Global 2000/The Carter Center; MAMSER (Mass Mobilization for Self-Reliance, Social Justice and Economic Recovery); DFRRI (Directorate of Food Roads and Rural Infrastructure); NYSC and Armed Forces.

Zonal Facilitators for each of the PHC quadrants were identified: Professor O. Kale (South West), Professor L.D. Edungbola (North West), Professor Eka Braide (South East), and Dr. M.K.O. Padonu (North East). Dr. Lola Sadiq was appointed as the National Coordinator.

1988: Memorandum of Understanding between Global 2000 and the Federal Government of Nigeria for the eradication of dracunculiasis was signed by President Jimmy Carter (for Global 2000) and Professor Olikoye Ransome-Kuti (for the Federal Government).

1988: Dracunculiasis was declared a reportable disease in Nigeria by the National Council on Health.

1988: Standardized forms and training guidelines were developed for use during the first National Case Search and using the WHO standard definition of a "case of dracunculiasis."

1988: State Task Forces for dracunculiasis eradication were inaugurated in Kwara, Katsina, Kaduna, Niger, Federal Capital Territory and Sokoto (Sokoto, Kebbi & Zamfara) States. His Eminence, the Sultan of Sokoto (Alh. Dr. Ibrahim Dasuki), attended the Sokoto Guinea Worn Task Force inauguration as his first official function after his installation.

1988: African Ministers of Health, under the auspices of the WHO, adopted the resolution to eradicate dracunculiasis in Africa by 1995. Professor Olikoye Ransome-Kuti (Hon. Minister of Health, Nigeria) co-sponsored the resolution.

1988: The Second African Regional Conference on Dracunculiasis Eradication was held in Accra, Ghana. The president of the host country (Flight Lieutenant Jerry Rawlings), the 39th President of the United States (President Jimmy Carter and his wife, Roselyn Carter), Professor G.L. Monekosso and Dr. Donald R. Hopkins attended the conference which was co-sponsored by WHO, UNICEF, UNDP, CDC (Atlanta), Global 2000, WASH (the Water, Sanitation and Hygiene project) and the Peace Corps (Benin).

The standard definition of a case of dracunculiasis was established and adopted globally.

1988:

- Dr. Donald R. Hopkins and Craig Withers, Jr. visited Kwara State, paid an advocacy visit to the Military Governor of the State (Group Captain Ibrahim Alkali), to the Hon. Commissioner for Health (Dr. Abdulkarim Ibrahim), to the Vice Chancellor (University of Ilorin, Professor Adeoye Adeniyi) and to the State Guinea Worm Task Force.
- Dr. Hopkins and his team visited Budo Ayan, a village in the State highly endemic for Guinea worm. The State Executives held a cocktail party in Government House in honor of the visitors.

1989: Independent Internal Evaluation of the first National Case Search was carried out by Professor O. Kale (Northern States) and Professor L.D. Edungbola (Souther States). The exercise led to greater coverage, more efficient case searching, and greater political commitment to interventions.

1989:

- Second National Conference on Dracunculiasis Eradication was convened.
- The results of the 1988/1989 second National Case Search were announced

1989:

- International Donors' Conference was held in Lagos Sheraton when the sum of US$10 million was realized for dracunculiasis eradication.
- The Carter Center (led by President Jimmy Carter and his wife), UNICEF, UNDP and the Federal Government of Nigeria sponsored the conference. UNDP Regional Director, Pierra-Claver Dambia, chaired the conference.
- His Eminence, the Sultan of Sokoto (Alh. Dr. Ibrahim Dasuki) and the Military Governor of Kwara State (Group Captain Ibrahim Alkali), attended the Donors' Conference. That was the first official function of the Sultan outside Sokoto State since his installation.

1990:

- Third National Conference on Dracunculiasis Eradication took place.
- The Federal Government declared March 20 of every year as Guinea Worm Day to strengthen dracunculiasis eradication activities, public enlightenment, advocacy and reporting.
- The results of the Third National Case Search (1989/1990) were announced.
- The Hon. Minister of Health (Professor Olikoye Ransome-Kuti) launched the Proceedings of Second National Conference on Dracunculiasis Eradication which was published as a supplement of the *Nigerian Journal of Parasitology* (Fig. 6.1).

1990: DuPont and Precision Fabrics donated a large quantity of monofilament nylon filters to Nigeria for dracunculiasis eradication, through the influence of The Carter Center.

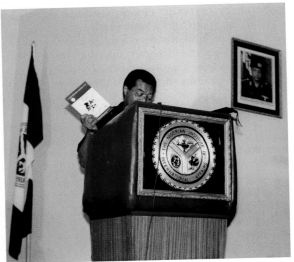

FIG. 6.1 The Hon. Minister of Health, Professor Olikoye Ransome-Kuti, launching the Proceedings of the Second National Conference on Dracunculiasis Elimination which was published as a supplement of the *Nigerian Journal of Parasitology* in 1995.

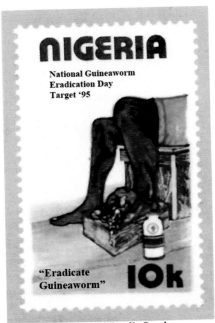

**Nigerian Philatelic Service.
First Day of issue was 20th March 1991.
(Stamp designed by G.N. Osuji)**

FIG. 6.2 Guinea Worm Disease Commemorative Postage Stamp.

1990: The Third African Regional Dracunculiasis Conference was held in Yamoussoukro, Cote d'Ivoire.

1991:

- The Fourth National Guinea Worm Conference took place and the First National Guinea Worm Day was observed.
- The results of the Fourth National Case Search (1990/1991) were released.
- The Federal Government of Nigeria demonstrated its commitment to dracunculiasis elimination in Nigeria when Vice-President Admiral Augustus Aikhomu unveiled three sets of commemorative postage stamps. A prototype is shown in Fig. 6.2.[2]
- The Vice-President also directed that all the 589 LGAs in 30 States and FCT should mandatorily devote 10% of their health budget to dracunculiasis eradication.
- The Federal Government urged national and international water projects to prioritize dracunculiasis endemic communities for rural water supplies.

1991: Creation of more States and LGAs to bring the figures to 30 (plus FCT) and 589, respectively. The creation of more States and LGAs was used advantageously by NIGEP to strengthen case searching, advocacy, grass roots participation and interventions.

1991: Village-based monthly surveillance commenced in full force, using standardized reporting forms, by village-based health workers, LGA supervisors and State Coordinators.

1991: A review of Ghanaian and Nigerian Guinea Worm Eradication Programs took place at The Carter Center, Atlanta, Georgia, USA under the chairmanship of the 39th US president, President Jimmy Carter and his wife, Rosalyn Carter (Fig. 6.3).

1991: The first meeting of managers of the Dracunculiasis Eradication Program was convened in Brazzaville under the sponsorship of the WHO (Afro), UNICEF, Global 2000 and the WHO Collaborating Center for the Eradication of Dracunculiasis. Professor G.L. Monekosso (WHO Regional Director) opened the conference.

1992: NIGEP functional zonal offices (secretariats) were created and empowered.

1992:

- The fourth African Regional Meeting of Managers was held in Enugu.

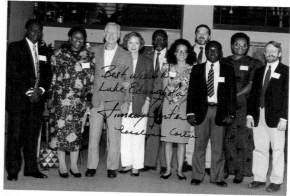

FIG. 6.3 President Jimmy Carter (chairman, The Carter Center) and his wife, Rosalynn Carter, with the NIGEP zonal facilitators and two Global 2000/The Carter Center technical advisors (Craig Withers Jr. and Pat McConnon) during the 1991 Ghana–Nigeria Program Review in Atlanta.

- President Jimmy Carter and his wife honored the NIGEP National Coordinator and zonal facilitators with awards of outstanding contribution to dracunculiasis eradication activities in Nigeria.
- President Jimmy Carter and his wife were also decorated with traditional titles in appreciation of their services to humanity (Fig. 6.4A).
- The First Lady, Mrs. Maryam Abacha, joined President Jimmy Carter and his wife in dracunculiasis eradication activities in some endemic villages (Fig. 6.4B).

1993: Case-containment intervention began.

1993: National Guinea Worm Day (March 20) was observed.

1993: Nigeria Guinea Eradication Program recorded a total 75,752 cases.

1993: Ethiopia hosted the Programme Review of Dracunculiasis Eradication Programs of English Speaking Endemic Countries (Ethiopia, Ghana, Kenya, Nigeria, Sudan and Uganda) which was sponsored by CDC, Global 2000 (The Carter Center), UNICEF, UNDP and WHO.

1994: National Task Force on Dracunculiasis Eradication was held in Sokoto. The opening ceremony was performed by the State Governor, Colonel Yakubu Mu'azu, and the Hon. Minister of Health, Dr. Dalhatu Sarki Tafida.

1995:

- The Eighth National Guinea Worm Conference took place and the Fifth National Guinea Worm Day was observed.
- NIGEP recorded a total of 16,374 cases in the year.

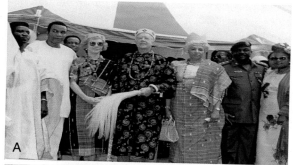

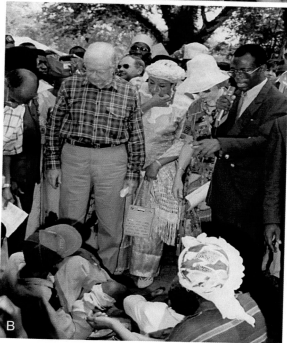

FIG. 6.4 **(A)** President Jimmy Carter (Chairman, The Carter Center) and his wife, Rosalynn Carter, traditionally decorated for their immense contributions toward the fight against Guinea worm disease. Mrs. Maryam Abacha (wife of Nigeria's former Head of State, General Sanni Abacha) is seen on the left of President Carter and Jim Nwobodo, former Governor of Enugu State, is on the right of Mrs. Carter. **(B)** President Jimmy Carter sympathizing with Guinea worm victims; Mrs. Maryam Abacha could not hold back her tears.

1995: Training of NIGEP field staff on vector control, using temephos (Abate) by Karl Kappus and his team from CDC, Atlanta, GA, USA.

1995: The 44th World Health Assembly initial target date for dracunculiasis eradication.

1995: Article on "Target date for the eradication of guinea worm disease: a reality or an illusion?" was published.[1]

1996: Creation of more States and LGAs to a national total of 36 States (plus the FCT) and 774 LGAs.

1996: The seventh National Guinea Worm Day was observed.

1996: Joint in-country evaluation of NIGEP activities by UNICEF, WHO, CDC (Atlanta), and Global 2000/The Carter Center.

1997: Program review meeting of the dracunculiasis eradication program in Ethiopia, Ghana, Kenya, Nigeria, Uganda, Sudan and Yemen. The meeting took place in the Sheraton Hotel, Sana'a, Yemen. The sponsors were The Carter Center (Global 2000), CDC, UNICEF and the WHO.

1998: The Ninth National Guinea Worm Day was observed.

1998: Dr. E.S. Miri was appointed the first Nigerian and the fifth Country Representative for Global 2000/The Carter Center in Nigeria.

1998: Mr. Craig Withers, Jr. visited the North West NIGEP zone and participated actively in field activities in Kwara, Niger, Kebbi and Zamfara States. Historically, on June 8, 1998, while working with Craig Withers Jr. in Nassarawa Melaiye, a hyperendemic village in Birnin Magaji LGA, Zamfara State, it was announced on the radio that the Head of State, General Abacha, had died.

1999: General Yakubu Gowon, former Nigeria Head of State and Chairman of the Board of Trustees of the Yakubu Gowon Center, partnered with The Carter Center to strengthen advocacy advantageously for dracunculiasis eradication in Nigeria.

1999: Cash rewards were introduced to strengthen surveillance and case reporting internally and across international borders.

1999: Zonal Facilitators for dracunculiasis eradication in Nigeria were redesignated as Zonal Consultants by The Carter Center.

1999: WHO established the International Certification Commission for Dracunculiasis Eradication.

2000: The Seventh Dracunculiasis Managers' Meeting was held in Sudan. Gen. Gowon, Professor A.B.C. Nwosu (Hon. Minister of Health), Dr. E.S. Miri, Zonal Consultants and NIGEP National Coordinator, attended the meeting.

2000: The 11th National Guinea Worm Day was observed.

2000: Resurgence of dracunculiasis in five villages in Dekina LGA, Kogi State after about 50 years after any previously known case.

2000: General Gowon advocacy visits to Kogi, Katsina and Zamfara States in the North West Zone of NIGEP.

2000: Extraordinary Zonal Debriefing on Dracunculiasis in Gusau, Zamfara State to launch a final onslaught on dracunculiasis in the North West Zone. The meeting led to the dramatic end of dracunculiasis in the zone.

2000: Zonal Taskforce Meeting on Dracunculiasis Eradication in Katsina State. Alh. Umaru Musa Yaradua (the Executive Governor of Katsina State, who eventually became Nigerian President) and General Yakubu Gowon, attended. Several boreholes and hand-dug wells were commissioned in the endemic villages as late as 8 p.m. (Fig. 6.5A−C).

2000: National Symposium on Dracunculiasis Eradication was organized at the Abuja Sheraton by the Federal Ministry of Health in collaboration with WHO, UNICEF, The Carter Center and Yakubu Gowon Centre. Guest speakers were General Yakubu Gowon, Professor Olikoye Ransome-Kuti and Professor L.D. Edungbola.

2000: An Extraordinary Zonal Task Force and Cross-Border Meeting with Niger Republic and Benin Republic were jointly held in Sokoto State. General Dr. Yakubu Gowon, the Executive Governor of Sokoto State (Alhaji Attahiru Dalhalu Bafarawa), Sokoto State Deputy Governor (Alh. Aliyu Magatakarda Wamakko), Dr. E.S. Miri, Dr. K.A. Ojodu, several commissioners, Directors, LGA Chairmen and the former Nigeria's High Commission to Great Britain, Alhaji Alhaji (the Sarduna of Sokoto), all attended the historic event. The highlight of the meeting was the commissioning of some 25 boreholes and several hand-dug wells by General Gowon and the State Executive Members. The exciting field work, which went on until 9 p.m., was "the last straw that dramatically broke the backbone of dracunculiasis in Sokoto State." (Fig. 6.6).

2001: Dracunculiasis Managers' Meeting was held in Lome, Togo. General Gowon attended with a sizable Nigerian contingent.

2002: The 13th National Guinea Worm Day was observed.

2002: Re-location, re-negotiation, and complete renovation (with water and electricity) of NIGEP's Zonal Office in Gusau, Zamfara State took place.

2002: The colorful commissioning of the impressively functioning integrated water supply to dracunculiasis endemic and high-risk communities by Prince Audu Abubarka, the Executive Governor of Kogi State, took place. The project was decisive for the elimination of dracunculiasis in the State and LGAs (Fig. 6.7A and B).

2002: The North West Zone conducted a comprehensive Internal Zonal Case Search in previously,

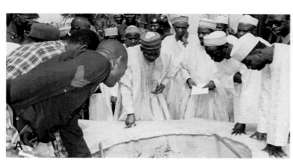
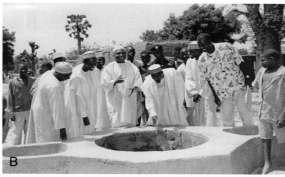
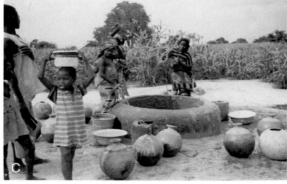

FIG. 6.5 **(A)** Former Head of State, General Dr. Yakubu Gowon, inspecting one of the new hand-dug wells in Karadua, Matazu LGA, Katsina State. **(B)** Dr. E.S. Miri (The Carter Center country representative) appreciating one of the hand-dug wells in the hyperendemic community of Karadua, Matazu LGA, Katsina State, following the effective intervention of Governor Musa Yar'Adua and the commissioning of several boreholes and hand-dug wells by General Dr. Yakubu Gowon and the Governor in the LGA. **(C)** A hand-dug well recently commissioned by General Dr. Yakubu Gowon at Karadua, Matazu LGA, Katsina State.

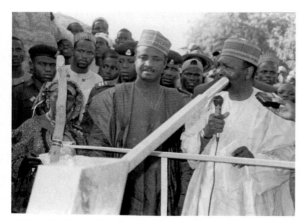

FIG. 6.6 General Dr. Yakubu Gowon, former Head of State (right) and His Excellency, Alh. Aliyu Magatakarda Wamakko, the Deputy Governor of Sokoto State (and the only Deputy Governor who served as chairman of the State Guinea Worm Taskforce) commissioning a new borehole in Tidi Bale, Isa LGA, Sokoto State.

recently and currently endemic States by LGA and village. The exercise strengthened advocacy for a safe water supply, maintenance and use; promoted sustained interventions and reporting and motivated total community participation.

2003: Joint review of the Sudan, Ghana, and Nigeria Dracunculiasis Eradication Program at The Carter Center, Atlanta, GA, USA.

2004:

- The 14th National Guinea Worm Day was observed.
- NIGEP recorded 495 case of dracunculiasis.
- September became the first month when no single case of dracunculiasis was recorded nationwide.

2005: Hon. Minister of Health, Professor Eyitayo Lambo, on behalf of President Olusegun Obasanjo, GCFR, inaugurated the National Certification Committee on Guinea Worm Disease Eradication with Professor A.B.O. Oyediran as the Chairman of the seven-member committee. The committee was

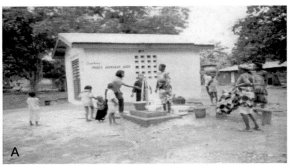

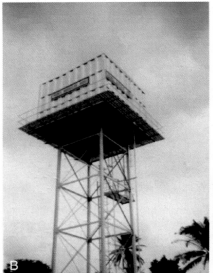

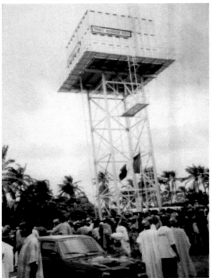

FIG. 6.7 **(A)** Borehole and engine house in Omadene from where water is being pumped into the overhead tank in Ajenejo. **(B)** Overhead tanks in Ajenjo, the most endemic village in Kogi State. Water in these tanks comes from the engine house shown in **(A)**.

strengthened by the co-option of the UN, non-government organizations and Ministry/Parastatals as nonstatutory members.

2006: NIGEP retrieved dracunculiasis data from the Carter Center in Jos to establish its own database at the NIGEP Secretariat in the Federal Ministry of Health, Abuja.

2007: The 17th National Guinea Worm Day was observed.

2008: The Eighth African Regional Managers' Meeting on Dracunculiasis Eradication was held in Abuja.

2008: The last case of dracunculiasis in Nigeria was recorded in Enugu State.

2009: General Dr. Yakubu Gowon was a special guest at the 20th National Guinea Worm Day.

2009: The first year with no case of dracunculiasis since the first National Conference on Dracunculiasis in Nigeria was convened about 25 years ago.

2009: The National Certification Committee on Guinea Worm Disease Eradication carried out Internal Evaluation of NIGEP activities. The North West Zone team conducted the exercise in 19 villages of nine LGAs in Kwara, Katsina, Kebi, Zamfara and Sokoto States.

2010: Evaluation of the interruption of the transmission cycle of indigenous dracunculiasis in Nigeria by an independent 13-member team of external and national evaluators sponsored by the WHO. The team included a WHO Consultant and a member of the International Certification Commission of Dracunculiasis Eradication (ICCDE).

2011: Nigeria received The Carter Center Award for dracunculiasis eradication after reporting no indigenous cases for more than two consecutive years. The award was made at the Carter Center, Atlanta, GA, USA, during the 15th Meeting of Programme Managers of Dracunculiasis Eradication.

2013: Nigeria was certified free of dracunculiasis by the WHO, having recorded no case for more than three consecutive years and, accordingly, recommended by WHO International Certification Commission.

2014: WHO presented the certificate to Nigeria as a **dracunculiasis-free country**.

REFERENCES

1. Edungbola LD, Ologe JO. The target date for the eradication of Guinea worm disease: a reality or an illusion? *Niger J Parasitol.* 1995;16:3−19.
2. Hopkins Dr, Hopkins EM. *Guineaworm: The End in Sight.* Chicago: Encyclopedia Britanica, Inc. Medical and Health Annual; 1992:10−27.

CHAPTER 7

Impact of Dracunculiasis (Guinea Worm Disease)

Dracunculiasis is not normally directly fatal but the public health impact of the disease is phenomenal, most especially on health, agriculture, education, socio-economic conditions and general development.

When uncomplicated, dracunculiasis causes relatively mild discomfort of limited duration. However, most cases are accompanied by secondary bacterial infection and complications arising from negligence, ignorance, poverty, poor personal hygiene, unhealthy methods of local management, multiple infections and the anatomic location of emerging worms at very delicate organs.

Under such conditions, dracunculiasis often becomes severely and permanently disabling, causing visual impairment and blindness,[19,3] complicated pregnancies,[15] sterility, abortion, paraplegia and quadriplegia,[1,7,9,12,18] constrictive pericarditis,[10] urinary obstruction,[17] osteomyelitis,[11] acute synovitis, ankylosis, arthritis and amputation.

Sometimes, myositosis develops, leading to chronic ulceration of bubo when the adult female worm ruptures in the body and releases numerous larvae in the tissue, causing large abscesses filled with pus.[6]

About 0.5% of Guinea worm victims experience permanent disability.[13] In Burkina Faso and Nigeria, dracunculiasis was established as the leading portal of entry and death by tetanus bacterial infection.[16]

The most well-documented quantitative reports on the impact of dracunculiasis morbidity are on agriculture and education. Muller[14] ranked dracunculiasis as the leading cause of protracted disability during the peak with regard to agricultural engagements among all diseases, including malaria.

The total annual wage loss and the global loss of marketable goods due to dracunculiasis has been estimated at US$170 million and US$300 million to US$1 billion, respectively.[20,8]

In 1987, Edungbola et al.[5] reported a loss of over US$20 million per year in profit from rice production alone due to endemic dracunculiasis in some rice-producing communities endemic for Guinea worm in South Eastern Nigeria with a population of about 1.6 million people. They also estimated that the cost of multiple interventions (safe water supply, health education, distribution of nylon monofilament filters, vector control, programs supporting communication plus sanitation) over a period of 5 years was about US$36 million, whereas the 45 million productive man-days lost (11.6% of total productive man-days lost) due to dracunculiasis per year was equivalent to about US$50 million worth of rice produced.

1. This analysis was based on rice alone. Yam, cassava, palm produce and soya beans are also produced and sold in large quantities.
2. Only a quarter of the land suitable for rice production had been used then. Thus, there was potential to expand rice production by at least 100%.
3. An additional 500,000–1,000,000 people could become actively involved in rice cultivation and some 20,000 direct jobs could be generated in the local rice-processing industries.

Several studies have shown that dracunculiasis accounts for about 33% of school absenteeism during the peak prevalence and ranked it as the leading cause of low school enrolment, poor academic performance, high dropout rates and delayed graduation.[4]

In addition, in endemic areas, dracunculiasis had been a major threat to social and religious observances, family stability and a significant constraint to the implementation of highly prioritized national and international programs, such as Primary Health Care, foods, roads, rural infrastructure, literacy program, breast feeding promotion, child survival, maternal welfare, malaria treatment and prevention, family planning, self-sufficiency in food production and security.[2]

Fig. 7.1 illustrates the adverse impact of dracunculiasis on health and the implementation of government policies and programs.

The Eradication of Dracunculiasis (Guinea Worm Disease) in Nigeria. https://doi.org/10.1016/B978-0-12-816764-9.00007-9

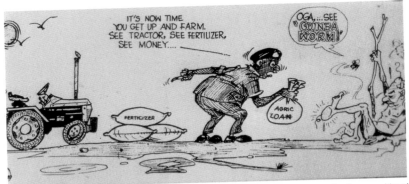

FIG. 7.1 A cartoon depicting the adverse impact of Guinea worm disease on agriculture and health. (Source: Daily Times, June 30, 1989.)

REFERENCES

1. Donaldson JR, Angelo TA. Quardriplegia due to Guinea worm. *J Bone Joint Surg*. 1961;43A:197—198.
2. Edungbola LD. *The Crawling Flier, the Flying Crawler, the Warring Worm and the Wormy World*. The 47th University of Ilorin Inaugural Lecture; 1995:120.
3. Edungbola LD, Adeleye MA. *Blindness Due to Ocular Dracunculiasis* (Unpublished). 2018.
4. Edungbola LD, Kale OO. Guineaworm disease. *Surgery*. 1991;98:2351—2354.
5. Edungbola LD, Braide EI, Nwosu AC, et al. *Guineaworm Control as a Major Contributor to Self-Sufficiency in Rice Production in Nigeria*. New York: United Nations Children's Fund; 1987. UNICEF/WATSAN/GW/2/87.
6. Fairley NH, Liston WG. Studies in the transmission of *Dracunculus medinensis*: a negative experiment. *Indian J Med Res*. 1924;12:93—103.
7. George JS. Bleeding in pregnancy due to retroplacenta situation of Guinea worm. *Ann Trop Med Parasitol*. 1972;69:383—386.
8. Golladay FL. Notes on economics of Dracunculiasis. In: *Proceedings of Workshop on Opportunities for Control of Dracunculiasis*. Washington, DC: National Research Council; June 16—19, 1982.
9. Khwaja MS, Jonathan FB, Dossertor JFB, Lawrie JHL. Extradural Guineaworm abscess. Report of two cases. *J Neurosurg*. 1975;43:627—630.
10. Kinare SG, Parrulkar GB, Sen PK. Constructive pericarditis resulting from dracunculiasis. *Br Med J*. 1962;1:845.
11. Mathur PPS, Dharker SR, Hian S, Sardana V. Lumbar extradural compression by Guineaworm infestation. *Surg Neurol*. 1982;17:127—129.
12. Mit AK, Haddock DRW. Paraplegia due to Guineaworm infection. *Trans R Soc Trop Med Hyg*. 1970;64:102—105.
13. Muller R. Dracunculus and Dracunculiasis. In: *Adv Parasitol*. 1971;9:73—140.
14. Muller R. Guineaworm disease; epidemiology, control and treatment. *Bull World Health Organ*. 1979;57(5):683—689.
15. Smith DJN, Siddique FH. Calcified guineaworm in the broad ligament of a pregnant mother. *J Obstetrics Gynecol Br Commonw*. 1965;72:808—809.
16. Primae U, Becquet R. Dracunculose et tétanos. A propos de 15 observations. *Bull Soc Pathol Exot*. 1963;56:469—474.
17. Raffi P, Dutz W. Urogenital dracunculiasis. Review of the literature and report of 3 cases. *J Urol*. 1967;97:542—545.
18. Reddy CRRM, Vasanta VV. Extradural Guineaworm abscess. *Am J Trop Med Hyg*. 1967;16:23—25.
19. Verma AK. Ocular dracunculiasis. *J Indian Med Assoc*. 1966;47:188.
20. Ward WB. The impact of dracunculiasis on the household. In: *Proceedings of Workshop on Opportunities for Control of Dracunculiasis*. Washington, DC: National Research Council; June 16—19, 1982.

c. "The ongoing drive to exterminate the Guinea worm is because of the money that people make by treating the humans they (Guinea worm) infect";
d. "The extermination campaign is because the Guinea worm is neither mega fauna nor photogenic like elephants, tigers, etc. and lacks advocates" and
e. "When the last Guinea worm is killed, the Earth's biodiversity will be irrevocably damaged."

General Comments:

- Guinea worm is a parasite that lives inside the human host from where it derives all the benefits and necessities of life and living to the detriment of the host who provides everything but gains nothing other than impoverishment, year after year, by adversely affecting and depleting health, education, agriculture, socioeconomic activities, general well-being and wholesome development. Smallpox and polio are diseases caused by viruses, just as dracunculiasis is caused by *Dracunculus medinensis* (a parasite).
- Guinea worm could have chosen to be free-living or be normal flora rather than being parasitic and depending absolutely on living in the tissues of man at his own grave disadvantage overall.

Fire could be naturally good and useful but when it starts to burn down houses or factories, under any circumstances, it is promptly extinguished to prevent further destructions.

When a tiger or lion escapes from the zoo cage and it starts killing people or threatening lives, the canine is killed without compromising its "mega fauna or photogenic" status with human life.

When a domestic dog becomes rabid and uncontrollably wild, it is exterminated because of the grave danger it poses to humans and other healthy animals.

- Most of the materials and resources being committed to the eradication of dracunculiasis are donated free of charge, largely because dracunculiasis has impoverished and depleted the endemic communities and countries of the necessary resources and initiatives to the extent that they cannot protect and save themselves on their own.
- **Who Is Responsible for the Crisis?**
  - (Asked by the **Save the Guinea Worm Foundation**)

Ironically and probably due to insufficient information or lack of knowledge, the Save the Guinea Worm Foundation is blaming or holding the following list of agencies responsible for an unnecessary cause because of their courage, sacrifices, humanitarian concerns, and determination to eradicate dracunculiasis.

Some of the agencies blacklisted by the Save the Guinea Worm Foundation include: the United Nations (WHO, UNICEF, UNDP, and World Bank and their international powerful agencies); the United States Agency for International Development; Centers for Disease Control and Prevention; The Carter Center (by inference) and the Bill Gates Foundation.

Should these agencies be blamed or commended and should the Save the Guinea Worm Foundation be commended, reprimanded or disapproved?

Conclusions

- It is most certain that proponents of the Save the Guinea Worm Foundation will change their minds when they see the suffering of a dracunculiasis victim with an emerging worm. They would be speechless and tender an unreserved apology if they saw a 25-year-old man with 84 emerging worms, a 2-year-old child with multiple infections, a pregnant woman with 36 fulminating attacks, an 80-year-old widow completely incapacitated, a disabled man wretchedly helpless or an orphan being tyrannized indiscriminately by the scourge of dracunculiasis, not just once in a life time but year after year for as long as they live in endemic communities without anyone coming to their rescue.
- Like a Nigerian proverb, it is true that "seeing is believing" but experience is the best teacher. A member of the Save the Guinea Worm Foundation who volunteered to be self-infected with Guinea worm will be in the position to tell the best story of what dracunculiasis is and whether or not it deserves to be protected (for the sake of enhancing biodiversity) or exterminated (for the sake of human dignity, well-being, and development). There seems to be some gaps in knowledge. Those opposing dracunculiasis eradication are apparently ignorant of what Guinea worm disease entails and its horrible impact in real life.
- All individuals, agency leaders and warriors who have remained undaunted in their unwavering battle against dracunculiasis (and thereby restoring human dignity), deserve congratulations and great commendations for a historic battle well fought, a victory well deserved and a mission well accomplished.

MISCELLANEOUS CHALLENGES

Some miscellaneous but equally serious impediments to the implementation of interventions include: the hiding of dracunculiasis cases; the hiding of unsafe sources of drinking water (pond) and the practice of unhealthy traditional management of dracunculiasis, (including the use of **Sekia** which often leads to serious complications, protracted incapacitation, permanent deformity or even death when accompanied by secondary bacterial infection).

Other miscellaneous challenges are:

1. Non-availability of the National Youth Service Corps (NYSC) due to incessant industrial action by the tertiary institutions in Nigeria. NYSC were the best source of staff recruitment for intervention and sustainability in dracunculiasis eradication;
2. Non-availability of petrol with its adverse consequences on mobility and field operations and
3. As beneficial as the use of external consultants can be, sometimes, probably due to lack of experience or

due to ignorance of the socio-cultural peculiarities and political sensitivity in the areas of operation, inflammatory comments often jeopardized the good relationship between the Nigerian field staff and their communities. This could be unhealthy, demoralizing, distracting and an important challenge in the control of tropical diseases.

REFERENCE

1. Save the Guinea Worm Foundation - Defending the world's most endangered species. www.deadlysins.com/guineaworm (Assessed 15th August, 2016).

CHAPTER 10

The Stagnation of Dracunculiasis Eradication in Nigeria (1996–99): Reality or a Mirage?

In 1991, the World Health Assembly adopted December 1995 as the target date for dracunculiasis eradication. At the expiration of the deadline, several African countries were still endemic (Fig. 10.1). Nigeria alone recorded 16,374 cases that year. By October 1996, a total of 129,903 cases had been reported to the World Health Organization (WHO) with about 100,000 (77%) cases coming exclusively from Sudan.[1]

As shown in Table 10.1, by the end of 1995, the number of Guinea worm cases in Nigeria had dropped to 16,374 (92%). However, from 1996 to 1999, the annual number of cases remained statistically the same, thereby, creating a "stagnation scare." Although the number of cases during the period of stagnancy remained perceivably unchanged, there was a phenomenal build up in re-strategizing, the introduction of new innovations, and a renewed determination and belief by all stakeholders that the eradication was not only achievable but in sight. These rapidly culminated in a dramatic drop in the number of cases to zero in 2009 and Nigeria was certified free of dracunculiasis in 2013.

The new innovations, re-strategizing and renewed determination that led to the dramatic drop in the number of cases include:

1. Unprecedented political commitment and action against dracunculiasis nationwide;
2. Massive public awareness and active societal participation in the eradication drive;
3. Training, empowerment and motivation of field staff to sharpen their skills for robust and sustained interventions;
4. Adequate provision, maintenance, and utilization of safe drinking water supplies, giving topmost priority to dracunculiasis endemic communities;
5. Reinvigoration of the administrative powerhouse of the Nigeria Guinea Worm Eradication Programme (NIGEP). Thus, Dr. E.S. Miri was appointed the Country Representative by The Carter Center, Zonal Facilitators were redesignated as Zonal Consultants by The Cater Center, an additional NIGEP zone was created and General Dr. Yakubu Gowon (Nigeria's former Head of State and President of the Yakubu

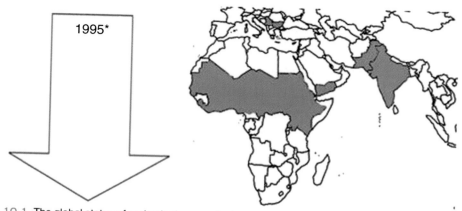

1995*

FIG. 10.1 The global status of endemic dracunculiasis at the 1995 target deadline for Guinea worm disease eradication.

TABLE 10.1
Selected Trends of Monthly Dracunculiasis Surveillance in Nigeria (1992–2009)

Trends	Year	No. of Cases
A. Dramatic reduction	1992	202,917
	1993	75,752
	1994	39,774
	1995	16,374
B. Stagnation	1996	12,282
	1997	12,590
	1998	13,419
	1999	13,247
C. Acceleration toward interruption of transmission	2000	7897
	2009	5355
	2002	3825
	2003	1459
	2004	495
	2005	120
	2006	16
	2007	73
	2008	38
D. Interruption of transmission and certification	2009–13	0
	2013	Certification by WHO

Modified from: Miri et al. (2010).[2]

Gowon Center) commenced partnership with the 39th President of the United States of America and Chairman of the Carter Center (Hon. Jimmy Carter and his wife) to implement very powerful and effective advocacy for dracunculiasis eradication in Nigeria;

6. The Federal Government, State Governments and Local Government Areas (LGAs) collaborated with The Carter Center, the United Nations Children's Fund, WHO, United Nations Development Programme, Japan International Cooperation Agency, and others to demonstrate an incredible commitment and support for dracunculiasis eradication at a level unprecedented in Nigeria;

7. The creation of more States (to 36 and the Federal Capital Territory) and more LGAs (to 774) enhanced greater accessibility to and coverage for surveillance, case detection and interventions in previously unreached or hard to reach endemic areas;

8. More resources and exposures, including funds, materials and participation in relevant meetings at zonal, national and international levels, became immensely advantageous and

9. Special interventions launched to accelerate the eradication campaign, including case containment, cash rewards, Guinea worm extraction, radical innovations, program integration, etc.

In conclusion, the period of the "stagnation scare" was a period of unperceivable progress when the primary focus and expectations were more on physical case reduction and not on the efforts expended in carefully and wholesomely putting all vital actions in place and launching a sustained final attack to make the resurgence and scourge of dracunculiasis an impossible reoccurrence.

The significant merits and benefits of the target date and the "stagnation scare" are that both encouraged the doubling of all efforts to accelerate the eradication drive rather than relaxing on the achievements that had been made, knowing too well that even a few remaining cases of active dracunculiasis could dangerously escalate the resurgence of the disease beyond imagination.

REFERENCES

1. World Health Organization. *Certification of Dracunculiasis Eradication: Criteria, Strategies, Procedures.* WHO/FIL/96/188; 1996.
2. Miri ES, Hopkins DR, Ruiz-Tiben, et al. Nigeria's Triumph: Dracunculiasis eradicated. *Am J Trop Med Hyg.* 2010;83: 215–225.

Nigeria Guinea Worm Eradication Programme (NIGEP): Evolution, Structure and Strategies

EVOLUTION

The chronological account of dracunculiasis in Nigeria has already been highlighted. In the early 1950s, researchers' attention was focused primarily on the copepods (water fleas) of the genus *Cyclops* which serves as the mandatory intermediate host of *Dracunculus mendinensis*, the etiologic agent of dracunculiasis. However, in the late 1970s, university researchers started to focus on the epidemiology and impact of dracunculiasis as well as bringing the problem to the attention of government officials, United Nations agencies and non-government organizations in Nigeria.

Multiple events, including the promotion of Primary Health Care, the Water Decade Declaration and the making of dracunculiasis eradication a World Health Organization (WHO) subgoal, the interest of the United Nations Children's Fund (UNICEF)/Rural Water and Sanitation Agency and the partnership of Global 2000 and The Carter Center with the Federal Government of Nigeria created the necessary momentum and impetus to make the dracunculiasis problem and its elimination a serious and highly prioritized national issue. When Professor Olikoye Ransome-Kuti was appointed the Hon. Minister of Health in 1986 by President I.B. Babangida (Grand Commander of the Order of the Federal Republic [GCFR]), he became a most valuable asset in convincing the Federal Government to commit to making dracunculiasis a reportable disease and a leading priority for eradication in Nigeria and Africa.

At that time, Nigeria had the highest number of cases of Guinea worm disease in the world (about 700,000 cases) and was not given a serious chance of success like Ghana, a neighboring country. However, with the dynamic leadership of Professor Olikoye Ransome-Kuti, the support of UNICEF and Global 2000 -The Carter Center, the unprecedented political commitment of the Federal Government of Nigeria and the overwhelming application of massive Nigerian's human resources to dracunculiasis eradication, Nigeria surprised the watching world and was certified free of dracunculiasis in 2013, even ahead of Ghana!

It is gratifying that at the onset, I had the privilege of interacting extensively with Mr. Richard S. Reid (UNICEF Country Representation in Nigeria), Professor Olikoye Ransome-Kuti (Hon. Minister of Health) and Dr. Donald R. Hopkins (Deputy Director at the Centers for Disease Control and Prevention [CDC], Atlanta, GA) on the prospect of dracunculiasis elimination in Nigeria.

In 1985, with the massive support of UNICEF (Nigeria) and in collaboration with CDC, Atlanta (through Dr. Donald R. Hopkins) and the University of Ilorin, the first National Conference on Dracunculiasis in Nigeria (the first of its kind in Africa) was held in Kwara Hotel, Ilorin, Kwara State, from March 25—27. During the conference, succinct national attention was drawn to the nationwide spread, impact and challenges of dracunculiasis and its elimination in Nigeria at a level far superior to what had ever been known in the country previously.

In 1987, UNICEF (Nigeria) sponsored a study to determine the impact of dracunculiasis on rice production in the rice bowl areas of South Eastern Nigeria (population 1.6 million). The results of the study were stunning and became important quantitative evidence to justify the impact and the elimination of Guinea worm disease.

The elimination drive in Nigeria became accelerated and on course in 1988 when the 39th President of the United States of America (Hon. Jimmy Carter and his wife) signed a Memorandum of Understanding, on behalf of Global 2000, with the Federal Government of Nigeria (represented by Professor Olikoye Ransome-Kuti, the Hon. Minister of Health).

In 1988, the maiden meeting of the ad hoc National Task Force (NTF) on Dracunculiasis Eradication in

The Eradication of Dracunculiasis (Guinea Worm Disease) in Nigeria. https://doi.org/10.1016/B978-0-12-816764-9.00011-0

Nigeria was held on May 5 and 6 in the Board Room of the Federal Epidemiological Unit, Onikan Health Center, Lagos.

The participants were: Dr. A.D. Kolawole (Chief Consultant, Epidemiological Unit, and the Chairman); Professor L.D. Edungbola; Dr. Eka Braide; Dr. C.N. Obionu (Anambra State Director of Health Services); Dr. M.K.O. Padonu; Dr. Lola Sadiq; Dr. O. Ogunnowo; Dr. B.B. Bhalerao (WHO) and Lloyd Donaldson (UNICEF, Nigeria).

In attendance were Dr. (Mrs.) O.O. Ojo, Dr. Y. Saka and Miss. E. Otok-Akpan. Professor O. Kale and Dr. Timi Agary (Federal Ministry of Science and Technology) were absent with apologies. Dr. Don. R. Hopkins (Senior Consultant, Global 2000) and Craig Withers, Jr. (the first Resident Technical Advisor for Global 2000) attended the second meeting on July 1, 1988.

Major decisions that emerged from the maiden meetings included:

1. Nigerian Guinea Worm Eradication Programme (NIGEP) will be adopted as the national nomenclature for the eradication drive;
2. The NIGEP secretariat will be based in the Federal Ministry of Health where all the eradication activities will be coordinated;
3. A multi-sectoral approach will be adopted for the planning and implementation of NIGEP activities;
4. Two national bodies, the NTF and the Steering committee, will spearhead the formation of national policy and the technical strategies, respectively, for NIGEP activities;
5. In addition to the NIGEP National Secretariat in the Federal Ministry of Health, NIGEP will be decentralized to four zones (North East, North West, South East, and South West) after the Zonal Structure for Primary Health Care quadrants (Fig. 11.1). Each of the four zones will be administratively and technically managed by a Zonal Facilitator (Dr. M.K.O. Padonu for North East, Professor L.D. Edungbola for North West, Dr. Eka Braide for South East and Professor O. Kale for South West). Dr. L.K. Sadiq was chosen as the National Coordinator of NIGEP;
6. The composition of the NTF of NIGEP was to be multi-sectoral and membership to include representative of the 22 States and Federal Capital Territory, Abuja and the Federal Ministries of Health, Agriculture, Education, Water Resources, Information, Science and Technology and the Armed Forces (Police and Immigration). Others included the Directorate of Food, Roads and Rural Infrastructure, Mass Mobilization for Socio-Economic Reform (MAMSER), National Youth Service Corps (NYSC), UNICEF, WHO,

United Nations Development Programme (UNDP) and Global 2000/Carter Center and
7. Membership of the Steering Committee to spearhead the technical strategies included the Director of Public Health & Disease Control (as the Chairman, representing the Hon. Minister of Health), Global 2000 Resident Technical Advisor (Co-Chairman), the NIGEP National Coordinator; the four Zonal Facilitators, the Federal Ministry of Water Resources, the Federal Ministry of Science and Technology, UNICEF, WHO and UNDP.

STRUCTURE

The revised organizational structure of NIGEP is shown in Table 11.1.

As a mandatory requirement to be certified free of dracunculiasis by the WHO International Certification Commission (ICC), after at least 3 consecutive years reporting zero cases (indication of interruption of transmission), Professor Eyitayo Lambo (the Hon. Minister of Health), on behalf of President Olusegun Obasanjo, GCFR, inaugurated the National Certification Committee on Guinea Worm Disease Eradication (NCC-GWDE) in 2005. The committee was chaired by Professor A.B.O. Oyediran (former Vice-Chancellor, University of Ibadan). Members of his committee were: Professor O. Kale; Professor L.D. Edungbola; Professor E.I. Braide; Professor A. Osibogun; Dr. A.P. Bassi and Mrs. I.N. Anagbogu (Secretary and NIGEP National Coordinator).

Federal Government Ministries/Departments/Agencies and Nongovernmental/UN Organizations co-opted onto the NCC-GWDE as non-statutory members included: the Ministries of Water Resources; Agriculture; Rural Development; Youth Development; Woman Affairs; Information and Communications; Science and Technology and the Primary Health Care Development Agency (PHCDA). Others were The Carter Center, WHO, UNICEF and The Yakubu Gowon Centre.

STRATEGIES

In general, integrated, multiple, multisectoral eradication strategies were adopted by NIGEP, based on the recommendations of the National Steering Committee and international dracunculiasis eradication formations. However, flexibilities in the adoption of specific strategies existed and other innovative interventions were used, depending on local peculiarities, such as religion, socio-cultural conditions, climatic disparities, rainfall pattern and variations in the period of the year when transmission occurs.

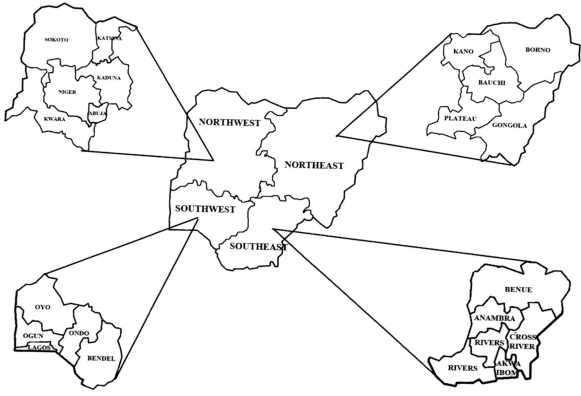

FIG. 11.1 The Zoning Structure the four Primary Health Care regions on which the operations of NIGEP were based in Nigeria at the onset in 1988.

For convenience, three different stages of targeted strategies are identifiable. These are: pre-intervention strategies; core intervention strategies and radical innovation strategies. Approaches and processes to pre-certification and free certification, are also distinct.

Pre-Intervention Strategies

These are largely: advocacy at local, national and international levels; public enlightenment and community mobilization; mobilization of resources and stakeholders; identification and training of manpower and fine-tuning of NIGEP structures (National Task Force, Steering Committee, Zonal Offices and task forces, state task forces and Active Case Searches).

Core Intervention Strategies

The main intervention strategies used are: adequate safe drinking water supply, utilization and maintenance; effective and sustained health education; fabrication, distribution, use and replacement of nylon monofilament filters and vector control, using temephos (Abate).

Other Intervention Strategies

These include:

1. Radical innovations (especially in the North West Zone but some were eventually adopted in other zones) using large-scale extraction of Guinea worms and case management; pond guards; the placing of filters, bowls, funnels and buckets at pond sites; town criers empowered with a megaphone; religious organization empowered with a megaphone; water and food hawkers; traditional rulers and healers; schools, markets and special festivals; nomadic associations; opinion leaders and politicians; promotion and distribution of free or affordable "Pure Water" sachets, especially during transmission and the translation of surveillance and health education materials into Ajamin (Hausa language written in Arabic) especially in the North West zone;
2. Case containment strategy;
3. Cash rewards;
4. The investigation of rumored cases;

TABLE 11.1
Organizational Structure of the Nigerian Guinea Worm Eradication Programme (1988–2009)

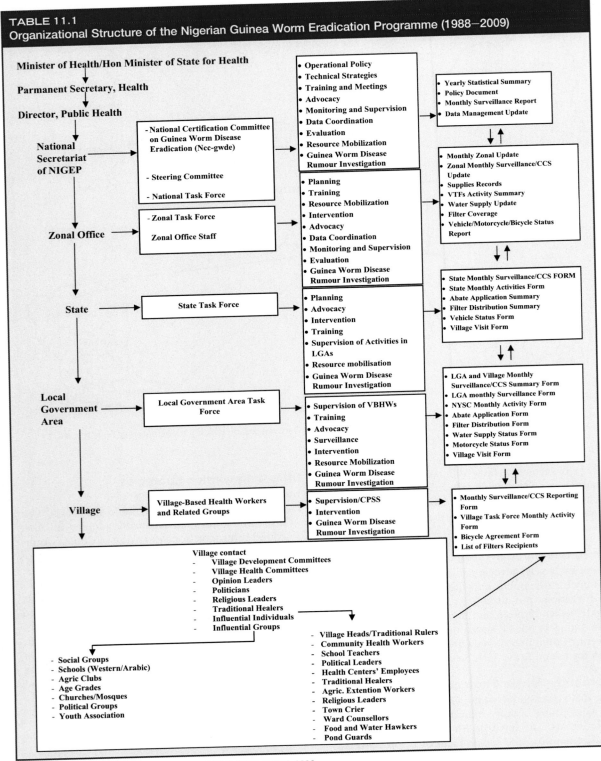

Revised from the First Interim Country Report NIGEP/NCC-GWDE, 2008.

5. Meetings, conferences, symposiums and technical review sessions and
6. Surveillance, monitoring, supervision and evaluation.

Certification Strategies/Processes
These featured three main events:

1. Formation of a National Certification Committee on Guinea Worm Disease Eradication (NCC-GWDE);
2. Assessment and recommendation by the Independent Certification Team after at least 3 consecutive years of zero case reporting and
3. Free Certification by the WHO International Certification Commission (ICC).

CHAPTER 12

Phenomenal But Real: Multiple Recountable Experiences During Dracunculiasis Elimination in Nigeria

DRACUNCULIASIS: A DISEASE OF MISPLACED PRIORITY?

In the earliest years of the establishment of the Faculty of Health Sciences, University of Ilorin, Ilorin, the preclinical classes in Epidemiology and Community Medicine and in the Community Based Experience and Services (COBES) postings were conducting demographic studies, disease inventory and need assessment surveys in a village located some 45 km away from Ilorin, the State Capital.

The village (population 750) had migrated down the hill (about 5 km) to resettle closer to the newly constructed North-South highway for better and more productive socio-economic opportunities. Whereas dracunculiasis was unknown at their old settlement site with a perennial stream, the new settlement with acute water scarcity, especially during the dry season, soon became endemic and notorious for dracunculiasis endemicity. Attempts to construct hand-dug wells were unsuccessful due to unfavorable hydrogeologic complications and lack of appropriate tools and technology.

During student-centered guided studies and during community focused group discussions, it was striking that the community prioritized having a secondary school and a court above having safe drinking water sources and other needs.

The villagers perceived a secondary school as a symbol of community prestige and the yearning for a court was to checkmate the rampart divorce of wives away from the village (because of the menace of Guinea worm infection year after year). It would be advantageous to the husband if the divorce case was tried in the husband's community and the opposite if her case was heard and determined in another court outside the husband's community.

Eventually, both projects were implemented but a few years later, dramatic events occurred. The secondary school was to be closed down because of unacceptable low enrolment, prolonged absenteeism due to Guinea worm infection and poor academic performance in public examinations, worsened by the refusal of qualified and committed teachers to be posted to the school because of the fear of dracunculiasis.

The pre-clinical students were to observe the village court session slated for assorted hearings, including divorce cases. Three consecutive court sittings could not be held because the magistrate himself was infected, incapacitated, and could not attend court sessions for months because of his Guinea worm disability. Arguably, the sustained endemicity of Guinea worm disease in this community could be rightly described as a disease of misplaced priority. However, with the United Nations Children's Fund (UNICEF) Assisted Rural Water Supply and Sanitation interventions in Kwara State in the late 1980s, dracunculiasis had since been eliminated in the village, in Kwara State and in Nigeria.

THE GUINEA WORM WITCHES

In 1989, during the evaluation of the third Active Case Search in the Southern States of Nigeria, Mr. Sanyaolu and I were stunned by what we encountered in a community (SP), in Ondo State.

On arrival, we met an uproar, a huge crowd and a masquerade decorated in fresh palm fronds and snail shells. The masquerade was accompanied by four guards with lashes and sticks in their hands (Fig. 12.1).

The masquerade, a chief priest and five traditional worshippers had just returned from the forest after 7 days of spiritual and ritual consultations to enquire from the ancestors what could be responsible for the worst community tragedy in 50 years (the unprecedented outbreak of Guinea worm disease!) No household, including those of the health center officials, in the community was spared. There was an average of five infected persons per household with protruding Guinea worm emerging from virtually all anatomic

The Eradication of Dracunculiasis (Guinea Worm Disease) in Nigeria. https://doi.org/10.1016/B978-0-12-816764-9.00012-2

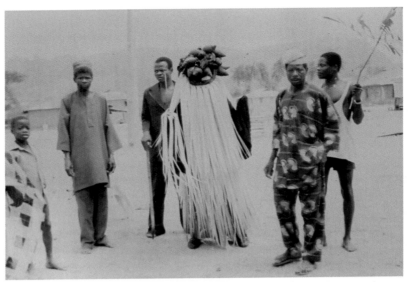

FIG. 12.1 The Guinea worm disease witches: a masquerade in SP going from house to house, picking the Guinea worm witches.

locations of the body. It was one of the worst and most severe outbreaks of dracunculiasis I had ever encountered!

When interviewed, the people freely, unanimously, and insistently implicated witches as the sole cause of the tragedy. The witches, harshly identified by the masquerade as he and his entourage moved from house to house, were severely and mercilessly beaten, disgraced and expelled from the community (to the embarrassment, shame and stigmatization of their children and relations). All the victims were elderly women (no single man was implicated). It was a most pathetic and highest manifestation of ignorance, taboos, traditional beliefs and abuse of women rights.

When we finally identified and met the community chief herbalist at his residence, we counted 17 cases of infected persons, mostly mentally derailed persons who the chief herbalist was treating for their mental derailments. The chief herbalist confidently confirmed that the outbreak was caused by witches as revealed by the oracle when ancestors were contacted. When asked if he knew the witches, the chief herbalist responded spontaneously and affirmatively. When asked why he allowed the witches to come and attack people in his house, he answered that he was traveling when the witches entered. We carefully put him through intensive health education on the cause, transmission, complications and prevention of Guinea worm disease. He was well educated and a retired civil servant.

It was striking that in that community, there was hardly any household without a graduate of a tertiary institution in virtually all major professions. At the end of health education and awareness promotions, the chief herbalist was excited, convinced and opened up on his past lifestyle. He brought out an old and disused aluminum jar with fitted porous filters. He informed us that when he was using it to filter his family drinking water, there was never a case of dracunculiasis in his household until the filter apparatus became dysfunctional. He eventually took us to the only community pond (an abandoned small dam) where everyone was obtaining drinking water by wading into it to fetch water. More importantly and fulfillingly, the chief herbalist voluntarily became our contact person who could be regarded as the first Village-Based Health Worker (VBHW) on dracunculiasis in Nigeria. He was giving, sustaining and enforcing health education messages, free of charge and voluntarily.

After those phenomenal encounters, we drove to Lagos (about 400 km away) to share these hard-to-believe experiences and horrors with Mr. Craig Withers, Jr., the new and first Global 2000 Resident Technical Advisor in Nigeria. He was emotionally touched but approved our initiatives. He promptly provided resources needed for immediate interventions as listed for him.

We hastily returned to Akure, the State capital, to mobilize the Director of Public Health and some of his staff for interventions. Also, we purchased case management needs and traveled back to the community. Ahead of our arrival, the chief herbalist (VBHW) had mobilized the people ready for intensive health education and case management.

Strikingly, because of the quality of interventions given, the regular follow-ups, the incredible efforts and commitment of the chief herbalist and the exceptional foresight of Ondo State for accepting and complying with beneficial packages (education, health, etc.), no indigenous case of dracunculiasis was seen in SP 2 years later and none since, until Nigeria was certified free of dracunculiasis by the World Health Organization (WHO) in 2013.

ARTIFICIAL GUINEA WORM

A similar but less dramatic experience occurred at about the same time in Gwagwalada, the most endemic Area Council in the Federal Capital Territory. During public awareness promotion, using audio-visual materials, one of the prominent traditional rulers and District Head attending the promotion demanded to know what to do about "artificial Guinea worm." To clarify his concern, he narrated a case of a witch woman (again no man was implicated) who was causing Guinea worm infections. When he was asked how he knew it was the woman, he responded that when the woman was arrested and beaten severely, she confessed that she was the cause of the Guinea worm outbreak. In-depth health education changed this erroneous belief that led to unjustifiable punishments inflicted on an innocent woman.

A YOUNG FARMER WITH UNPRECEDENTED 84 EMERGING GUINEA WORMS!

Arguably, a world record-setting but most pathetic encounter, which ended dramatically as a most celebrated attraction that came to the attention of Nigeria's former Head of State (Gen. Dr. Yakubu Gowon), The Carter Center, the Nigeria Guinea Worm Eradication Programme (NIGEP) and international reporters from Atlanta, Georgia, USA, was a case of a 24-year-old farmer (Rb) from whom 84 Guinea worms were extracted in Krg village, Dustsima LGA, Katsina State, during a single transmission season.

When found, the victim (Fig. 12.2), a bachelor, was severely emaciated and anemic, manifesting the characteristic symptoms of dracunculiasis toxemia.

Because of his condition, appropriate nutritional interventions were given first, including rehydration, before the extraction of his "legion" of Guinea worms. During the extraction, he was also managed for secondary bacterial infections and the risk of complications, including tetanus. He was monitored and given follow-up treatments and replenished with fortified nourishment for about 10 days. He recovered completely and dramatically!

Two years later, he was revisited. Gen. Dr. Yakubu Gowon was especially interested in Rb's case. Seeing is

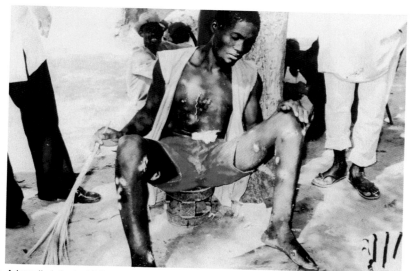

FIG. 12.2 A heavily infected 24-year-old farmer from whose body 84 emerging adult female Guinea worms were recovered in a single transmission year.

believing! On arrival in Krg (Rb's village), it was by coincidence that we met a large crowd in his compound. He was being traditionally decorated and celebrated as the best farmer and harvester of the year in that community. He had also married two wives and one of the wives had a set of twins, both boys! He had also bought a brand new motor cycle.

What a dramatic demonstration and justification of the investment in and commitment to dracunculiasis eradication and what a transformation from sickness to wellness, from poverty to prosperity, from obscurity and neglect to edification and celebration and from being a victim to being a victor!

It is gratifying that Rb became a most resourceful local person in dracunculiasis eradication by using his newly uplifted social status and personal experience:

1. To mobilize Guinea worm victims for timely self-reporting (even before the worm emerges);
2. To abolish the use of **Sekia** (a dangerous traditional practice of treating dracunculiasis);
3. To promote the observance of health education messages (including the avoidance of contaminating drinking water sources) and
4. To mobilize communities for safe water supply and maintenance, jointly with local, national and international water providers.

HIS EXCELLENCY, PRESIDENT ALHAJI UMARU MUSA YAR'ADUA LED THE SUCCESSFUL WAR AGAINST DRACUNCULIASIS (GUINEA WORM DISEASE)

When he was serving as the Executive Governor of Katsina State, just before he became the President and Commander-in-Chief of the Armed Forces of the Federal Republic of Nigeria, His Excellency, Alhaji Umaru Musa Yar'Adua, gallantly led and fought Guinea worm disease to elimination in Karadua, Matazu LGA in Katsina State.

The outbreak was so unprecedentedly severe in the community and Local Government Areas (LGA) that socioeconomic activities, during that rainy season, were completely paralyzed. Farmers, housewives, and children were bedridden. Schools were closed down because of incapacitation of infected pupils and teachers. NIGEP (North West Zone)/The Carter Center staff immediately launched aggressive interventions, including massive health education, distribution of nylon monofilament filters, vector control (using temephos [Abate]) and large-scale extraction of Guinea worms.

However, long-term permanent interventions, including concerted political commitment to prevent future outbreaks, were absolutely necessary. In conjunction with the Chairman of the Health Committee of the State House of Assembly, NIGEP/The Carter Center in the zone mobilized the National Television Authority (NTA) to cover and show the alarming outbreak sensationally on television.

The program was shown on NTA Katsina, immediately after the State news. The Chairman of the Health Committee was with the Executive Governor when the Guinea worm outbreak was beamed on the State NTA. He called the attention of the Executive Governor to the horror of human devastation caused by indiscriminate attack of villagers by Guinea worm disease.

The humane Governor was emotionally disturbed and speechless. When he was told the community being featured on the TV and the interventions that the NIGEP/The Carter Center staff were giving, he instructed the Chairman of the State House of Assembly Health Committee and I to be at Government House by 6.30 a.m. the following morning.

Promptly at 6.30 a.m., with his driver, the three of us headed to Karadua village in Malazu LGA. The State Commissioner of Police followed when he found out that the Executive Governor was passing through the Police Barracks along the high way.

At Karadua, His Excellency was exceedingly sad and visibly shaken when he saw many infected victims and witnessed the extraction and management of many cases by the surgical extraction and management team of S. Olukade, A. Sanyaolu, E. Edungbola and L. Ajileye of the NIGEP North West Zone. The Governor also went from house to house, assessing the horror of the adversity and sympathizing with the victims.

After consulting with the NIGEP/The Carter Center team and the Chairman of the Health Committee on what should be done and knowing that health education and provision of safe drinking water were the permanent solutions, he took the following steps:

1. That funds should be released immediately to UNICEF/RUWATSAN in Kaduna to sink boreholes in all the endemic villages within 2 weeks;
2. Personally donated the sum of ₦400,000 to the LGA for the welfare of the victims, including food;
3. Directed that healthy young men and migrant farm laborers should be hired to assist on the farms of infected farmers, because it was the peak time for agricultural activities;
4. His Excellency personally gave health education and instructed that infected persons should not enter drinking water ponds to avoid contaminating it and spreading the infection and

5. He informed the community that they should comply with all the health education and other interventions that the NIGEP/The Carter Center staff were giving.

Within 2 weeks, using two drilling rigs and operating on two shifts, all day and all night, several boreholes (by UNICEF) and hand-dug wells (by the United Nations Development Programme [UNDP]/LGA) had been provided in Karadua and in all other endemic communities in the LGA.

To coincide with the Zonal Task Force Meeting, which took place in Kastina and where His Excellency, Alhaji Umaru Muas Yar'Adua, was the Special Guest of Honor (Fig. 12.3A and B), General Dr. Yakubu Gowon, the former Head of State and President of the Yakubu Gowon Centre, was invited to commission several boreholes and hand-dug wells in Matazu LGA and in some other LGAs from 9.00 a.m. to about 8.00 p.m.

The former Head of State was accompanied by members of the State Executive Council, members of the State House of Assembly, Chairmen of LGAs, The Carter Center Country Representative, NIGEP National Coordinator, UNICEF, UNDP and participants from the 9 States in the North West Zone who were attending the Zonal Task Force meeting in Katsina.

During the January–December 1999 transmission season, 207 cases of dracunculiasis were recorded in Karadua village alone, ranking it as the most endemic village of the 225 endemic villages in the NIGEP North West Zone. By December 2000, only three cases were recorded i.e., a drop of 99%!

Within 3 years, transmission of Guinea worm disease had been interrupted in Matazu LGA. The elimination of the disease in Katsina State was accelerated and accomplished well before Nigeria was officially certified free of dracunculiasis in 2013.

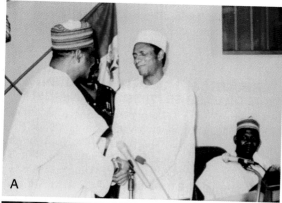

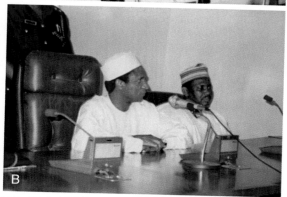

FIG. 12.3 NIGEP North West Zone Task Force Meeting in Katsina State in 2000. **(A)** Gen. Dr. Yakubu Gowon and His Excellency, Alh. Umaru Musa Yar'adua (the Executive Governor of Katsina State) exchanging pleasantries during the meeting. **(B)** Governor Umaru Musa Yar'adua, the Special Guest of Honor, addressing the participants.

THE ELIMINATION OF DRACUNCULIASIS IN KOGI STATE: REMARKABLE POLITICAL AND PUBLIC HEALTH LESSONS

Kogi State was one of the few States in Nigeria to be given Guinea worm disease-free certificates by the Federal Ministry of Health/NIGEP in 1995 to symbolize the initial target date for dracunculiasis eradication.

No case of dracunculiasis was known in the Dekina LGA of Kogi State in the past 50 years, including when the States was part of the old Kwara State. Alarmingly, during the 2000/2001 transmission season, 88 cases of the disease were confirmed in Dekina LGA, ranking the LGA the third most endemic LGA among the 37 endemic LGAs in the NIGEP North West Zone during that period.

There was widespread pandemonium in the LGA. Some elderly people associated the unknown disease outbreak to the anger of their ancestors while others attributed it to ivermectin (Mectizan) which was recently distributed for the prevention and control of River blindness.

In view of the vulnerability of Kogi State (sharing boundaries with 11 States, most of which were highly endemic for Guinea worms), NIGEP/The Carter Center North West Zone moved swiftly under the supervision of Dr. Job Adewunmi and Mr. Solomon Olukade to launch aggressive interventions. These included: establishing the magnitude and spread of the problem; promotion of effective health education; application of vector control, using temephos (Abate); distribution of nylon monofilament filters to all individuals by household; large-scale surgical extraction of Guinea worms and comprehensive case management.

Notwithstanding those interventions, the risk of potential yearly outbreaks remained considerable because the provision and use of safe drinking water was the fastest, most permanent, and most cost-effective strategy for the elimination of Guinea worm disease. In this regard, UNICEF/RUWATSAN in the State and the Directorate of Rural Development were the most promising water providers in the State.

However, the timely provision of safe drinking water to endemic and high-risk communities demanded prompt political attention and commitment at the highest level. Thus, high-profile advocacy by Gen. Dr. Yakubu Gowon (former Nigeria Head of State) was sought. Although the advocacy made substantial impact, the pace of implementation was adversely slow. The propensity of dracunculiasis to establish and disseminate rapidly demanded urgent action.

While considering possible effective solutions, I became determined to see and speak directly with the Executive Governor. Luckily, I succeeded, through the Hon. Commissioner for Health, a Veterinary Doctor and an in-law of His Excellency. The discussion was brief. I genuinely commended the Governor for his innovative projects, including: the State University; the Confluence Hotel; Housing Projects; Road Constructions and the elegant Presidential Lodge. As His Excellency was expressing (in body language) his appreciation and personal satisfaction about my commendations, I was quick to add that to the "outside world" dracunculiasis endemicity in an area connotes underdevelopment and poor leadership. As the governor winked, I repeated my last remarks. I was humbled when His Excellency asked, "then, Professor, what are we to do?" I politely responded that safe drinking water (boreholes and/or hand-dug wells) was the quickest, most permanent, and most cost-effective intervention to eliminate dracunculiasis in record time.

In my presence, His Excellency sent for Alhaji Alfa Ibn Mustafa, the Director General (Directorate of Rural Development in Kogi State) and mandated him to ensure immediate provision of sustainable safe drinking water to the affected villages. As I was joyfully and satisfactorily taking my leave, the Executive Governor requested that Gen. Dr. Yakubu Gowon should come to commission the water project in 4 weeks.

His Excellency fulfilled his promise. A most elegant water project was completed in timely fashion. Large quantities of borehole assorted spare parts were procured for future use when the need arises. Also,

two community pump maintenance artisans were employed and trained for each village.

Although Gen. Dr. Yakubu Gowon was out of the country and could not attend the commissioning, the ceremony was colorful, with a large crowd thrilled by a display of traditional celebrations by assorted groups of masquerades (Fig. 12.4A—C.)

After 2 years, no single case of Guinea worm disease was recorded and transmission was permanently interrupted before Nigeria was certified free of dracunculiasis in 2013 by the WHO.

His Excellency, Prince Abubakar Audu, the Executive Governor of Kogi State, died about a decade later, sadly on the day he was to be declared the elected Executive Governor of Kogi State again. However, the legacy of his contributions, especially in the elimination of dracunculiasis in Kogi State, remains arguably an unsung but most significant, phenomenal and memorable achievement. Strikingly, Nigeria was certified free of dracunculiasis by the WHO in the lifetime of Prince Abubakar Audu, the erstwhile and flamboyant Executive Governor of Kogi State. May his soul rest in perfect peace.

INTERPOLITICAL HOSTILITY BUT GUINEA WORM DISEASE SETTLED THE ANIMOSITY

The Chairman of a LGA hyperendemic for Guinea worm disease, in the newly created Zamfara State (by General Sanni Abacha), in the NIGEP North West Zone, enthusiastically demonstrated political will and commitment to dracunculiasis elimination in his new LGA. He procured 15,000 filters and distributed them to every household in the endemic villages. More importantly, he embarked on providing safe drinking water (boreholes and hand-dug wells) to the endemic communities. He did not exclude the most endemic village in the LGA (which coincidentally was the home town of his political rival) from enjoying all interventions for dracunculiasis elimination. His political rival did not reciprocate positively instead, it was alleged that he was deliberately damaging and rendering the boreholes non-functional in his own community and in the neighboring villages.

Under a new dispensation, the intolerant rival was controversially declared the winner and the Chief Executive of the LGA. The outgoing Chairman did not contend the questionable outcome of the election. Not long after, the new victorious Chairman was not reporting in his office. He was incapacitated by multiple Guinea worm infections. His wife and three children were similarly infected and bed-ridden.

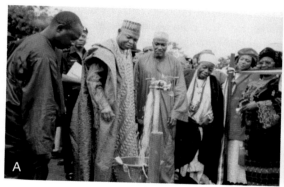
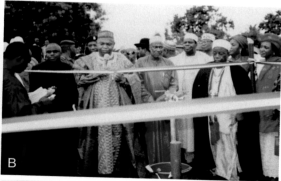
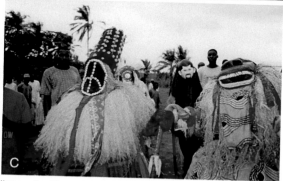

FIG. 12.4 **(A)** His Excellency, the Executive Governor of Kogi State, Prince Audu Abubakar, commissioning the Safe Water Project in five hyperendemic villages in Dekina LGA, Kogi State. **(B)** Governor Prince Audu Abubakar commissioning one of several boreholes in Dekina LGA. **(C)** Masquerades entertaining a huge crowd during the celebrated commissioning of the integrated Safe Water Supply in the five hyperendemic villages in Dekina LGA, Kogi State, in 2002.

The pathetic condition of the new Chief Executive and his family was brought to our attention. The NIGEP surgical Guinea worm extraction team was directed to attend to the incapacitated family in an hotel in Gusau, the State capital. The family had been transferred to the hotel from the village. In addition to surgical extraction of their worms, they were also given comprehensive treatment (wound washing and antiseptic dressings) to manage their secondary bacterial infections and prevent tetanus complications. They all recovered dramatically. The new LGA Chief Executive became very remorseful of his misdeeds and became supportive of the eradication drive.

That was how Guinea worm disease settled the score and reconciled the new Chairman with the humanitarian activities of NIGEP/The Carter Center in the North West Zone.

THE MIRACLE THAT BURIED GUINEA WORM DISEASE ALIVE!

The Modomawa Dam was a massive lake of water, which was impounded in the early 1980s by the former President, Alhaji Shehu Shagari, to address the acute problem of water scarcity in the locality. The dam was situated in the Birnin Magaji LGA in the newly created Zamfara State (by the late Gen. Sani Abacha, then Nigerian Military Head of State). Although the dam was a blessing in providing water for all domestic activities, animals, irrigation and water-hawking business, it became a persistent source of hyperendemicity, transmission and dissemination of Guinea worm disease.

Although very aggressive interventions, including: advocacy; surveillance; health education; filter distribution and assorted radical innovations were mounted, the impact was limited. It became necessary to embark on vector control, using temephos (Abate) to kill the cyclops (the intermediate host of the Guinea worm). The vector control strategy had not been used because of the large volume of water in the lake. It took an eight-man team of NIGEP/The Carter Center staff (plus the assistance of volunteered villagers) 2 days to technically determine the volume of water to be treated in order to calculate the quantity of temephos to be added for effective treatment of the dam.

After determining the volume of temephos to use, it usually took the team (again with the assistance of village volunteers) a whole day to effectively apply the chemical to the lake. This cumbersome procedure had to be repeated twice every month! On one occasion and as usual, the volume of the water and the quantity of temephos to apply had been determined. Drums of the chemical were kept ready on the banks of the lake for use the following day. At 6.30 a.m. on the treatment day, the team left Gusau (the State Capital) for Modomowa. On arrival at the dam, we were flabbergasted, stunned, and bewildered by what we saw. An incredible miracle had occurred! The massive volume of water in the Modomawa Dam had disappeared! YES, completely vanished, leaving only fish, amphibians (frogs and toads), aquatic insects and water plants bare on the wet slippery water bed! Joyfully, no case of Guinea worm disease was recorded in the community after 2 years and none before the WHO certified Nigeria free of dracunculiasis in 2013!

Some experts believed that a "land/mud slide" was responsible for the miraculous vanishing of water from the dam. Several eyewitnesses believed that it was a miracle by the hands of the Almighty God who mercifully ended the perennial pains and agonies of Guinea worm disease and the elimination efforts. As an additional benefit of the water vanishing from the dam, the incident accelerated the provision of safe drinking water (boreholes and hand-dug wells) to the affected communities.

GUINEA WORM IN THE STATE HOUSE OF ASSEMBLY

One of the core strategies that led to the elimination of dracunculiasis in Nigeria was vector control, using temephos (Abate), a safe chemical that selectively kill cyclops (water fleas), the intermediate host of the Guinea worm. Without cyclops, there will be no Guinea worm disease!

The American Cyanamid Co. was the world's exclusive manufacturer of the Abate chemical. In 1990, the company donated, through The Carter Center, enough Abate for use until the eradication of dracunculiasis was achieved in Nigeria and in all endemic countries. Although Abate was safe and used at a very low concentration (only 2 ml added to a 1 cm^3 of pond water), its use led to a significant reduction in the number of Guinea worm cases in endemic communities where the product had been used in this State (SS) and in

Nigeria generally. However, after a while, there were insinuations that pond water treated with Abate was polluting the water and rendering it unusable for ablution. Strikingly, no adverse effects of the chemical on humans, animals, or plants had occurred. Also, pond water treated with the chemical remained colorless, tasteless and odorless.

Through the State Director of Public Health who doubled up as the Chairman of the State Taskforce on Dracunculiasis Eradication, I was invited (as The Carter Center Zonal Consultant) to make some clarifications to the State House of Assembly on the concerns about the suitability and acceptability of water being treated with Abate for ablution.

With advanced privilege information, I had prepared slides to show the horror of dracunculiasis in the State. I had also prepared pond water containing several live cyclops, a small quantity of Abate and a dissecting microscope mounted with a relatively large screen (courtesy of UNICEF, Nigeria). The members of the State House of Assembly (most were from areas endemic for Guinea worm disease) were not hostile but gently and maturely presented the concern of the people (especially the religious leaders) about the effect of Abate on the suitability of pond water treated with it for ablution.

Having thanked the Honorable Members and obtained permission, I first made a slide presentation of the pathetic conditions of several men, women, and children infected with multiple Guinea worms, which were emerging from different parts of their bodies. I then proceeded with demonstration using the dissecting microscopes with the mounted screen.

The first demonstration showed live fast-swimming cyclops and some other aquatic organisms on the screen. Honorable Members were all silent. For the second demonstration, I added a drop of Abate to the petri dish containing the live cyclops. In less than 2 min, the cyclops were all motionless and dead. Some were enlarged and shown on the screen to reveal the structures of a cyclop and some associated aquatic organisms. The third demonstration was pond water free of any living cyclops after the pond had been treated for 4—8 h.

After the demonstrations, the silent House applauded with a loud ovation. There, in our presence, members unanimously adopted the resolution that Abate was safe and that it actually made water cleaner, purer, more hygienic and better for ablution than the raw pond water with cyclops, assorted insects, strange plants, and unknown small water creatures. This was a big boost for dracunculiasis elimination interventions as the House advised all LGAs not only to support the treatment of ponds with Abate but also to comply with health education messages and to prioritize the provision of safe drinking water to villages endemic for Guinea worm disease.

AN OUTBREAK OF DRACUNCULIASIS FOLLOWING THE BREAKDOWN OF A PASSENGER TRAIN: A STRIKING PANORAMA OF EVENTS

Until the late 1970s, dracunculiasis (Guinea worm disease) was unknown in Budo Ayan, a community located some 60 km from Ilorin (the Kwara State Capital). According to the Village Head and his subjects, Guinea worm disease first appeared in the community some months after a North-South-bound passenger train broke down on the outskirts of the community. Stranded passengers invaded the village for food, water, and personal needs. They remained dependent on the village for 5 days. The villagers affirmed that they noticed thread-like worms on the legs of some passengers who were seen performing ablutions in and around the only community pond. They also insisted that those passengers introduced the infection into their water.

The Village Besieged by Guinea Worm Disease

Due to ignorance of the cause, source, and prevention of the disease and since everyone was drinking from the same pond, dracunculiasis rapidly became highly endemic. No household was spared the attack annually. Men, women and children were indiscriminately infected. Several farmers were incapacitated and bedridden for months. Most of the Primary School pupils, including the head boy and the headmaster, were infected and could not attend classes for several weeks. Social events, including marriages were cancelled because either the bride or the groom or both were infected and incapacitated for months. Some could not fulfil their religious aspirations of undertaking a holy pilgrimage to Mecca and Medina because the emergence of their worms coincided with the time of air-lifting to the Holy Land.

Thus, dracunculiasis had paralyzed agricultural, educational, sociocultural, religious, and economic activities in the village. Some natives who were traders in Lagos and other bigger towns were brought back to the village when their worms emerged. These were indigenes who had come home for weddings, religious festivals and other community events during the dry season when transmission was ongoing.

During our first house-to-house community case search, we recorded an 88% infection rate. Multiple infections and disease complications were common, mostly due to unhygienic conditions and unhealthy traditional methods of managing the infected persons. Children were not spared. Weeping and wailing were heard in virtually all the houses as the traditional healer went from house to house, using his red-hot iron instrument, to puncture Guinea worm swellings and ulcers (Fig. 12.5A and B).

As a result of secondary bacterial infection and the resulting complications, we found a middle-aged man who was a successful business man in Lagos but had been brought to the village because of his Guinea worm infection. He claimed that he had spent all he had, including selling his clothes and goats to pay the traditional healers and spiritualists. His leg had to be amputated in the Teaching Hospital and donations collected to buy him crutches (Fig. 12.6). There was also an old woman with swollen and complicated knee (Fig. 12.7A and B). Her leg was also eventually amputated because secondary bacterial complications had become a threat to her life.

Absolute Water Scarcity

Water scarcity in the village during a dry season had become so severe that drinking water, while eating, had to be rationed in the family. At community level, scooping oozing water had to be on a rotation basis by household. It had also become mandatory for the few men who could manage to go out or whose worms had not yet emerged to go out early every morning to dig a marshy area (Fig. 12.8) until enough water oozed out for scooping before it was depleted.

No Water to Wash a New Set of Twins

It was most pathetic that during my follow-up visit to the village on a weekend, my attention was drawn to a young housewife (sent home from Lagos) who just delivered a set of twins. That was her first delivery. However, there was no water to wash the babies. The small quantity available was dark brown and muddy. It was a common practice by indigenes in Lagos and other big towns to send their pregnant wives to the village to deliver their babies in the belief that the older women in the village were better birth attendants for better and safer delivery. On seeing the helpless situation to wash and clean the new twins, I drove back to Ilorin, bought four 50-L plastic jericans, filled them with treated water behind my office in the Teaching Hospital and drove back to the village.

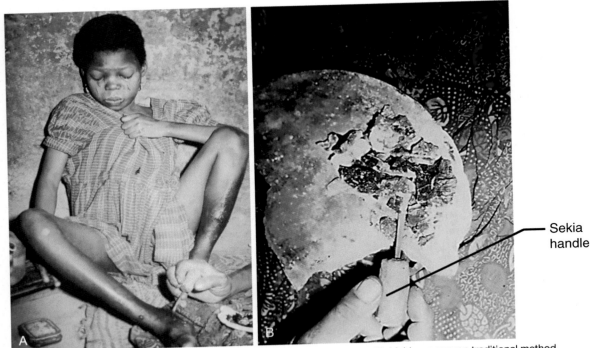

FIG. 12.5 **(A)** Puncturing a Guinea worm abscess with a red-hot iron (**Sekia**) is a common traditional method of management which invariably leads to serious complications. **(B)** **Sekia** is being heated to redness in hot charcoals.

I requested the family and birth attendants to bring some storage containers to receive the water which had "become gold" in the language of the village head. One of the containers brought was a big metal bowl that was white on the inside. As we started pouring the water into the bowl (several observers had gathered under a tree to watch), a young boy, about 8 years old (with his two hands on his head; Fig. 12.9) shouted "E wo b'omi se mo!" (see how clean water is!). Truly, he had never seen such clean colorless water! Dr. Don Hopkins later queried "what Primary Health Care is if a boy does not know what clean water looks like"!

We continued to supply 200 L of water weekly until the mother and her twins returned to Lagos.

Telefest

The peak of a severe outbreak of dracunculiasis in Budo Ayan coincided with the Telefest competition when all the NTA Stations nationwide competed for the best presentation. NTA Ilorin, under Vickie Olumidi as the Station Manager and her team, made a presentation on "Dracunculiasis in Budo Ayan." Several things happened thereafter:

1. NTA Ilorin "Dracunculiasis in Budo Ayan", came second nationally, narrowly missing the first prize by a point;

2. When indigenes of Budo Ayan in Lagos and in other cities saw the program and their people incapacitated by Guinea worms on the TV, they were embarrassed, sad and furious, hurrying back to the village to confirm what they saw on the national TV.

3. **Home coming and safe water provision**
   The coming home of indigenes from Lagos and other big towns provided an opportunity for a community meeting and enough money was raised, in collaboration with UNICEF and Kwara State Government to provide safe drinking water sources (boreholes and hand-dug wells). Also, intense and sustained health education on the transmission and prevention of dracunculiasis was given;

4. **Guinea worm disease is no more!**
   Within 3 years, the transmission of Guinea worm-disease had been interrupted and the disease never reappeared in the community before Nigeria was certified free of dracunculiasis in 2013 by the WHO.

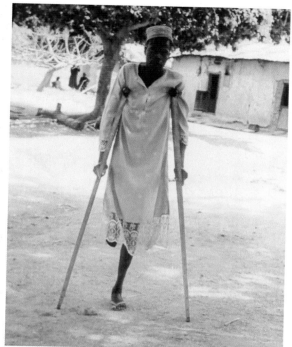

FIG. 12.6 A Lagos-based business man who suffered severe multiple Guinea worm infections. The right leg had to be amputated due to complicated secondary bacterial infection to save his life.

5. **Twenty-five years later**
   In 2009, during the Independent Internal Evaluation of NIGEP by the National Certification Committee of Guinea Worm Disease Eradication (NCCG-WDE) as mandated by the WHO, we visited Budo Ayan. The people were apprehensive and suspicious of our presence (amid the waves of insecurity that were prevailing in the country).
   As the community leaders were asking who we were, one of them who arrived a bit later said "E o ranti Dr. Edungbola?" (can't you remember Dr. Edungbola?). That was 25 years later! It was a great moment of emotional fulfilment for me that dracunculiasis had been eliminated in the village besieged by Guinea worm disease, causing much havoc;

6. **Children and teenagers do not know about Guinea worms 25 years later**
   Following the elimination of dracunculiasis in the community, a secondary school was established in the area. Our evaluation team interviewed several male and female students if they knew what Guinea worm was. All the answers were "E mi o mo o" (me, I don't know), except a boy who said he knew what

Guinea worm was. He brought a village boy with ring worm (a fungal infection) on his head! All the students born in the past 20 years did not know what a Guinea worm was!;

7. **Guinea worm baby?**
   As we were assessing an old borehole, a woman came with a boy who had finished Senior Secondary three (SS3) and told us that at the time the borehole was drilled, she had five Guinea worms emerging from her body and that she was carrying the pregnancy of the boy and.

8. **Death of Guinea worm disease celebrated**
   The oldest woman in the community was overjoyed about the elimination of dracunculiasis in the village. She disclosed that there was virtually no year she did not suffer a Guinea worm infection. She entertained us by what she called a "Guinea worm elimination dance."

A COMMUNITY WHERE GUINEA WORM DISEASE INFECTED ONLY MEN BUT WHY?

Characteristically, in endemic villages, Guinea worm disease does not discriminate who it attacks. Anyone (male, female, adult, child, indigene or visitor) who drinks water contaminated by an infected person will almost certainly experience the emergence of Guinea worm on his/her body about a year later.

During a religious festival, some 40 men had left their non-endemic village for Yankaba (an hyperendemic community) for celebrations. The two communities are separated by a lake. Because a water transport system does not exist, people traveling between the two villages (only about 3 kilometers apart) have to travel about 12 km on land (passing through Sabon Garin and Kaura Namoda).

Yankaba, a highly endemic village, is about 5 km from Kaura Nammoda, an important railway terminus in Zamfara State, in the North West. By coincidence, on the day of the celebration of the religious festival, the NIGEP/The Carter Center teams were carrying out dracunculiasis intervention (health education, filter distribution, vector control, borehole re-functioning, surgical extraction of Guinea worms and comprehensive case management). The team met the religious leaders at the ceremony and warned the participants not to drink untreated water in the community because of the ongoing transmission of dracunculiasis in the community. Filters were given to all the participants and the usage of the filters was demonstrated. About a year later, the LGA Guinea worm Coordinator came to NIGEP/The Carter Center to report an outbreak of dracunculiasis in a new village.

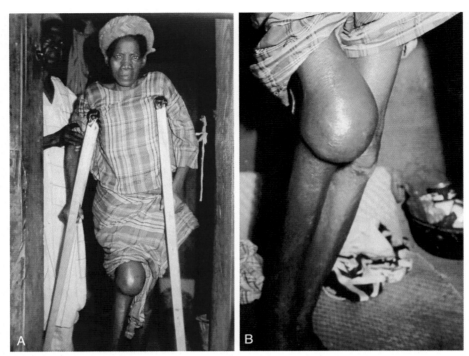

FIG. 12.7 **(A** and **B)** An elderly woman with severe synovitis on her right knee due to dracunculiasis. The leg was eventually amputated to save her life.

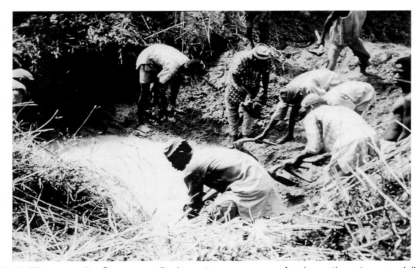

FIG. 12.8 Water scarcity: Some men digging out swampy areas for domestic water on a daily basis.

It was striking that all the people infected in that village were adult males. No single case occurred among the women and children. Our investigation revealed that all the infected individuals were those who went to Yankaba a year before for the festival. Of the 40 men who went, only six were not infected. The six admitted that they did not drink water in Yankaba because of the warning we gave them.

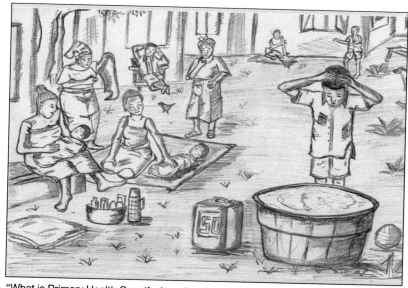

FIG. 12.9 "What is Primary Health Care if a boy does not know what clean water looks like?" -Don Hopkins.

The NIGEP/The Carter Center Staff launched holistic interventions: house-to-house case searching; a total health education package; treatment of all available ponds in the community with temephos to kill the cyclops; filter distribution and extraction of all pre-emerging and emerging worms. A Guinea worm Field Manager (Halimat) was assigned to the community exclusively, a VBHW was identified and empowered, advocacy for safe water supply was mounted at the LGA, State, and community levels, and intermittent visits were carried out by NIGEP/The Carter Center Senior Staff. No single case of dracunculiasis was recorded a year later and none thereafter before Nigeria was certified free of dracunculiasis by the WHO in 2013.

DRACUNCULIASIS OUTBREAK WITHOUT ENDEMICITY

Social functions, including multiple weddings, funeral events, Sallah celebrations, and graduation activities occur most commonly during the Christmas-New Year seasons and during the first quarters of the new year in Kwara State and in other parts of Nigeria. That period coincides with the dry season and favorable weather for mass outdoor activities and celebrations. Also, during that period, Kwara State indigenes doing business in Lagos, Ibadan, Ilorin, Osogbo, Kaduna and other cities and big towns usually come home to visit and celebrate with their families and other relatives in the village.

On this particular occasion, as usual, several indigenes of a community (located less than 20 km from the Kwara State Capital) had arrived home from Lagos and other places of businesses. Because of the large number of the people in the village that year for various celebrations, water scarcity was a limiting factor. Bottled and sacheted water were virtually unknown then. To meet the water demands of a large number of people, commercial water tankers supplied drinking water into drums and large plastic tanks for domestic consumption and other uses.

Normally, commercial water tankers were expected to obtain their treated drinkable water supplies from the State Water Cooperation. However, probably due to ignorance, his own convenience, or his commercial interests, this supplier was going to a nearby village (with a broken-down community dam) to fill his tanks free of charge. Unfortunately, the community where he was obtaining his free water was hyperendemic for Guinea worm disease and the broken-down dam was the exclusive site of transmission year in year out.

Unknown to the villagers, visitors, and celebrants, heavily contaminated water was indiscriminately consumed raw and untreated (neither boiled or filtered). A year later, when the incubation period of Guinea worm disease had lapsed, at least 18 Lagos-based business men, women and some children who had previously visited their native community during celebrations the previous year had Guinea worms emerging on different parts of their bodies. Most of the victims were brought to the village for treatment.

The report of an outbreak in that community was made to a joint Guinea worm team of the University of Ilorin and Kwara State Epidemiology Unit. At that time, NIGEP had not been constituted but UNICEF-RUWATSAN was at an advanced stage of commencing operations in Kwara State. An investigation revealed that all the infected persons in the village and from Lagos (32 altogether) were in the village the previous year and remembered drinking from the water supplied by the commercial water tanker. Also, it was confirmed that the vendor of the commercial water tanker obtained the water he supplied from the community dam where Guinea worm transmission was occurring. However, he denied knowing that the dam was infested with Guinea worm.

An epidemiological visit to the village, jointly with the late Dr. Adeleye (the Chief State Epidemiologist), revealed that the community (from where the drinking water was collected) was so hyperendemic for dracunculiasis that the community secondary school was virtually closed down because of perennial outbreaks of Guinea worm disease and incapacitation and because of the students' deplorable performance in their West African School Certificate Examinations. Also, during our visit, we saw one of the worst and most pathetic cases of Guinea worm disease, a 35-year-old man with a Guinea worm emerging from his left eye!

Thereafter, massive health education was given to the two communities involved, a large number of locally fabricated baft-cloth filters were distributed, Solomon Olukade, Dr. J.O. Idowu and the nurses of the Public Health Division extracted the Guinea worms and provided comprehensive case management. UNICEF-RUWATSAN (KwS) eventually provided safe drinking water sources (boreholes) to the affected communities.

It is gratifying that the transmission of Guinea worm disease had been interrupted in both communities and in all other endemic villages in Kwara State, even before Nigeria was officially certified free of dracunculiasis by the WHO in 2013. Today, indigenes of previously endemic villages can freely and safely come home to celebrate Christmas, New Year, Sallah, marriages and other festivals without the fear of Guinea worm disease. It is equally gratifying that agricultural, health, educational, religious, political and socio-economic activities have attained an unprecedented boost since the elimination of dracunculiasis in these two communities and in all others.

COMMERCIALIZATION OF GUINEA WORM DISEASE?

At the onset of the UNICEF-RUWATSAN take-off in Kwara State, villages endemic for Guinea worm disease were prioritized for safe drinking water supply (boreholes). A major obstacle encountered in the implementation of that laudable gesture was the reluctance and outright refusal of the villagers to use the newly provided safe water sources which would prevent the transmission of Guinea worm disease. The villagers preferred their Guinea worm-infested pond water for two main reasons-

1. Because their ancestors will be offended and a grave calamity would ensue if the natural ponds were abandoned for borehole water and
2. Because borehole water had a strange and an unpleasant taste.

Although health education campaigns were intensified, breaking the traditional beliefs and taboos remained a major challenge for a while.

However, as the drilling of boreholes continued in Asa and Moro LGAs under Harry Abe (the Project Manager), the State Hon. Commissioner for Health (Dr. Abdulkarim Ibrahim), his Director General of Health (Alh. Olayiwola Kamaldeen), and the Hon Commissioner for Local Government and Rural Development (Alh. Adamu Gene) were leading health education campaigns while Solomon Olukade, Dr. J.R. Idowu, and the nurses of the Public Health Section were carrying out effective Guinea worm extraction and case management. All those activities were receiving unprecedented political backing by the Military Governor of Kwara State, Group Captain Ibrahim Alkali. Those efforts paid off and the number of cases of dracunculiasis dropped dramatically in endemic communities that willingly participated.

As the impact became noticeable and the news spread, many more villages were self-reporting that their communities were endemic for Guinea worm disease and that they were eligible to get boreholes. In the process of confirming the self-reports of endemic status, we visited a village that had no case of Guinea worm disease in our record of a recent case search. However, the village head had reported 36 cases. Although people were presented for worm extraction and case management during the verification visit, we observed that all the victims presented to us in the village had recently been seen in other endemic neighboring villages. Further investigations revealed that all the cases presented were "imported" from other villages endemic for Guinea worm for an incentive fee of ₦300 per recruited patient, excluding free transportation.

That was how borehole water became acceptable and in high demands both in endemic and non-endemic villages because, like Guinea worm disease, water scarcity, especially during the dry season, was a formidable challenge in most villages and towns.

Although water scarcity still remains a major problem, the effectiveness of safe water sources provided by UNICEF-RUWATSAN, the European Union, Niger River Basin, DFRRI, private hand-dug wells and boreholes and the advent of bottled and sacheted water, have been advantageous in eliminating dracunculiasis, in reducing water-borne, water-associated and water-related diseases and in reducing the perennial scarcity of safe drinking water.

CHAPTER 13

In the Jaws of Death: Six Gruesome Encounters During Dracunculiasis Elimination in Nigeria

Dracunculiasis eradication activities were a prolonged fierce battle, excruciatingly demanding and unimaginably hazardous with attendant incessant exposures to infectious diseases, insecurity, insurgencies, mishaps, psychologic trauma and extreme deprivation. Luckily, over a period of more than two decades, we recorded only one death of a Senior Zonal Staff member during active service.

Aside from the unexaggerated experiences of my zonal staff and other colleagues, I personally encountered four very intimidating and life-threatening armed robbery attacks. During two of those confrontations, my official field vehicles were snatched at gun point and several vital and irreplaceable official and personal items were taken away, leaving behind the scars of the battle against Guinea worm disease as permanent memories.

Amidst all the dangers encountered, the Lord kept his covenants and remained faithful to his promises. Thus, when we passed through the waters, He was with us; through the rivers, we did not drown; when we walked through fire, we were neither burned nor scorched by the flames!

There were many undocumented but gruesome experiences, testimonies, encounters, hostilities, adverse sentiments, harassments and personal losses that cannot be accommodated in this book. However, a few of my personal encounters, while "in the jaws of death," are highlighted in this section as examples of life-threatening adversities and grave dangers that were encountered during the dracunculiasis eradication battle, with emphasis on the experiences in the North West Zone of the Nigerian Guinea Worm Eradication Programme (NIGEP).

Hopefully, these encounters and experiences will serve as warnings and reminders of the need for awareness of the intimidating challenges and dangers that are inevitable in the fight against tropical diseases and promotion of public health initiatives.

THE FIRST BAPTISM OF THE CHALLENGES DURING DRACUNCULIASIS ELIMINATION

Before NIGEP was launched in 1988, the University of Ilorin had actively been involved in dracunculiasis eradication initiatives through: the COBES program; training curricula in pathological sciences, epidemiology and community health and through collaborative research among members of staff in the Faculties of Health Sciences, Business & Social Sciences, Arts and Education.

The efforts and commitment were so impressive that the United Nations Children's Fund (UNICEF Nigeria) donated a Toyota Land Cruiser to strengthen related field activities that included active case searches (in Asa and in the neighboring Igbon community in Oyo State), the promotion of public awareness on the transmission, prevention, and control of Guinea worm disease (using Radio Kwara, Nigeria Television Authority, and the newspapers) and mobilization of self and community reporting of cases.

On one fateful day, a team of field assistants, medical students and researchers had been assigned and conveyed to specific villages, in groups of three and four, for Guinea worm field activities. The only vehicle available was the recently donated UNICEF Land Cruiser. I was to drive the participants to their assigned villages and collect them, in turns, when they had finished. I was to start collecting the field workers from Igbon, the most distant community, and then pick up the others from villages along the Ogbomosho-Ilorin highway. On approaching Igbon Day Secondary School where the field assistants were waiting for me, having observed the relevant highway rules and driving ethics, I was making a left turn from the main road when a recklessly speeding driver of a Peugeot 505 emerged from nowhere and crashed against the left side of my vehicle. The Land Cruiser somersaulted twice, throwing me out through the boot! During the horrifying crash, I could remember

The Eradication of Dracunculiasis (Guinea Worm Disease) in Nigeria. https://doi.org/10.1016/B978-0-12-816764-9.00013-4

saying "**the Blood of Jesus Christ**." Fortunately, I escaped virtually unhurt physically but the Land Cruiser was badly damaged with the laminated tinted windscreen completely smashed. At the police station in Ogbomoso, it was discovered that the driver could not produce his driver's license He was sent to Ilorin but drove to Jebba instead (an additional distance of 200 km) for his own personal undertakings. That was the reason for his extreme recklessness as he tried to make up for the time he had expended on going the extra kilometers. Although the Land Cruiser was repaired by the boss of the offending driver, this took considerable time and caused some delays in our field activities.

That unpleasant tragedy heralded the impending challenges, obstacles and hazards ahead and cautioned us to be vigilant, careful and ready to make sacrifices in the fierce, justifiable but promising battle against dracunculiasis.

THE KANKIA FLOOD: SUBMERGED BUT NOT DROWNED

The field trip started early and smoothly from Katsina, after purchasing plastic waste baskets and disposable polythene bags for delivery to the Guinea worm extracting team who were working in hyperendemic rural villages in Kankia, Katsina State, on that day. At X village, the unexpected happened. A journey scheduled to take a maximum of 1 h took more than 10 h. In a dry deep sandy river gully, just outside the village, our Land Cruiser sank into the sandy river bed. There were two of us, the driver and myself, but I drove. The auxiliary gear failed. In the process of waiting while mobilizing assistance from the villagers (it was during Ramadan), an amazing flood rushed down from upstream. There was no rainfall at our location at that time. With incredible rapidity, the flood almost covered the Land Cruiser, making it to drift slowly downstream. There was not enough time to evacuate all perishable items and intervention materials from the vehicle (Fig. 13.1A and B).

About 9 h later, when the villagers were breaking their fast, the flood had subsided considerably and villagers could cross the deep and sandy river bed from one side to the other. Several villagers had gathered, most as spectators, but some had the necessary rescue experience to tackle our predicament. They brought long strong ropes and tied them to the vehicle to pull it up the river bed. Unfortunately, the vehicle could only be pulled in the opposite direction to where we wanted to go. After about 45 min, the vehicle was successfully pulled up the sloppy and slippery bank to the shore. Water, sand, and other debris had filled the

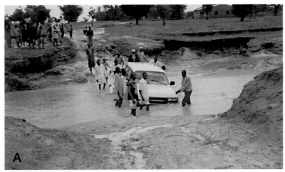

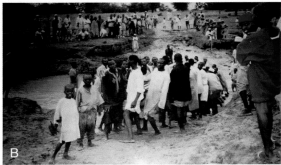

FIG. 13.1 **(A)** The Kankia flood that buried my NIGEP/The Carter Center Land Cruiser. The water had receded but there were too few helping hands to help with rescue until after breaking of their fast at 7 p.m. **(B)** After breaking their Ramadan fast, many more volunteers gathered around the vehicle to help pull it out, on a very slippery road, after being stranded for about 10 h.

engine and other hollow parts of the vehicle. There were two very experienced village drivers among the rescue volunteers. One took the key from me and after massive pushing by a large crowd, the engine started successfully. The driver used the accelerator to blow out water and sand from the engine. It took another 30 min to make a U-turn and to point the vehicle in the return direction. After thanking the villagers, they warned that I should not stop the engine during our journey of a distance of 10 km to the main Dutsima-Kankia road, another 15 km to Kankia, and 60 km to Katsina (85km in all)!.

Alas! The most dreadful episode had just begun! That journey was probably the greatest adventure of my life. Between the village where we were rescued and the main Dutsima-Kankia road (about 10 km), there was a long narrow bridge with no hand rail or demarcation to show the edge of the bridge on either side. When we were crossing it in the morning, we passed over it, driving very cautiously. However,

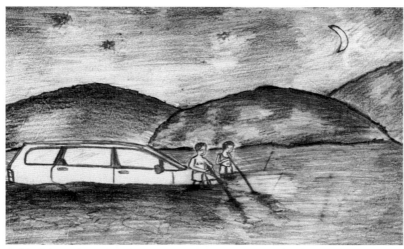

FIG. 13.2 Guided by two boys in the bright moonlight to drive over a long unseen bridge completely covered by rain floods.

by the time we got there on our return at about 9.30 p.m., the entire area had been flooded with rain water. The bridge had also been completely covered and was not visible. We dare not stop otherwise the roaring flood could wash away the vehicle to an unknown destination. I was prepared for the worst but remained prayerful. Miraculously, two young boys appeared from nowhere, apparently trying to collect fish that had been washed ashore by the flood. The boys tried to locate and show me the edges of the bridge (completely covered with water), using the sticks in their hands. Prayerfully, I positioned one boy at the right edge of the unseen bridge and the second boy at the other edge. I instructed them to move gently, using their long sticks, to mark the edges of the submerged bridge as they moved like a blind person trying to find his way (Fig. 13.2). I drove very carefully between the two boys, nervously but prayerfully. After about 15 min, we got to the other side of the bridge and on land!. I gladly compensated the boys with some money, two plastic buckets and bowls, some filters, soaked bread, and some biscuits.

At Kankia, we woke up the Guinea worm extraction team in their hotel and shared our experience with them before quickly proceeding to Katsina (60 km away). By God's grace and mercy, we arrived in Liyafa Hotel, in Katsina, at about 1.30 a.m.

Early in the morning, a motor mechanic worked on the vehicle, blowing sand, debris, and water out of the engine and other parts of the vehicle. At about 2.00 p.m., the mechanic had finished the work. On the way back to Ilorin to prepare the monthly report,

the vehicle stopped at about 4 km from Kankara. I took public transport to call on a motor mechanic who followed me with a towing vehicle and provided me with accommodation and food because there was no hotel. They worked on the engine the following morning and concluded that it had "knocked". The only option was to go to Kano, about 2 hours drive, to purchase spare parts for the engine because I did not have enough money to buy a new engine. After 3 days, the work was completed. We managed to drive the vehicle to Ilorin before the engine packed up again. However, very timely, Dr. E.S. Miri, The Carter Center Country Representative, bought a new engine to replace the damaged one because it was during the peak of rainy season transmission when about 90% of Guinea worm cases occurred in the zone. This experience was one of my most hazardous encounters during dracunculiasis eradication and in my life. The experience reveals the greatness of God, His grace, His compassion and His capability to make a way out of no way and to send help amidst helpless situations!.

THE GUINEA WORM "MERCENARIES": PROPERTIES FOR LIFE

The eradication of dracunculiasis was a fierce battle, directly against the disease and indirectly against its unhired and opportunistic "mercenaries." Although human casualties were limited, considerable properties were lost and psychologic trauma was immeasurable. However, the end justified the means!

A typical case, among several others, was the attack by armed robbers at the Jebba Toll Gate on the way to Niger State, during the peak of transmission in the North West NIGEP Zone and shortly after Nigeria's former Head of State, Gen. Dr. Yakubu Gowon, made an advocacy visit to Niger State. At the officially unmanned toll gate, just after the Jebba Bridge on the River Niger and outside the ancient town of Jebba where monuments to Mongo Park are found, a car drove close to our new Toyota Hilux provided by The Carter Center and waved us down. The lead attacker came out smiling and pretending to be a familiar friend and like someone who wanted to report an outbreak of Guinea worm. The general public had been enlightened to report such outbreaks. Our Hilux was loaded with assorted intervention materials, salaries to pay field staff in the zone, and personal property. Two of the assailants jumped into the Hilux, seized the key from the ignition, pushed the driver out, and pointed a gun at me. In unanticipated shock, I told them that we were members of the Guinea worm eradication team. The gunman pointed his gun at me again, threatening to shoot but the gang leader quickly commanded him not to. I pleaded that they should allow me to take my bunch of keys. They ignored my request, pushed me out and drove away in the direction of Ilorin while their own vehicle, with the two other members of the gang, followed them. This was the second vehicle snatching I encountered at gun point.

It was a traumatic experience because none of the uniformed officials in the vicinity or the petty traders could help. Besides, the vehicle and all the property in it were gone, untraceable, except for the mystery of a photograph of Guinea worm disease that was in an album in my bag that was stolen with the snatched Toyota Hilux. A few years after the attack, I came across the photograph somewhere but no one could account for its source.

What mixed feelings! The vehicle was stolen, valuable properties lost and dracunculiasis eradicated but the deep scars of the psychological trauma caused by the tragedy remain a relapsing and dreadful memory.

THE KAFANCHAN MAYHEM AND THE UNCOMMON FAVORS

By divine intervention, on a most dreadful day of extreme hostility, violence, fire, arson, blood and killings, death was apparently put to sleep for the staff of NIGEP North West Zone. While travelling to Jos to submit monthly reports and to collect intervention materials for the North West Zone during the peak of dracunculiasis transmission, my driver and I arrived at Kafanchan via the Jere-Kowi-Kafanchan road at about 9.00 p.m. We were not aware that deadly violence, marred by wanton destructions of life and properties, had just occurred at Kafanchan and a dusk to dawn curfew had been imposed on the commercial town. While wondering why the town was so deserted, smoky, and dead-silent, a group of stern looking and fully armed uniformed soldiers confronted us, aggressively demanding to know who we were. Having confirmed that we were NIGEP/The Carter Center staff on Guinea worm eradication assignment, they wondered why we were endangering our lives at that place and time. After rebuking us for our own sake and safety, the commanding officer ordered four fully armed soldiers to escort us safely out of the Kafanchan town to Kagoro-Akwanga Junction.

It was frightening that night to drive through the deserted and silent smoldering town. We saw several razed buildings, vehicles, locally made weapons, and some dead bodies by the road side. In sincere appreciation of the uncommon favor shown to us by the Nigerian soldiers that night, we offered our rescuers a token amount in gratification. Surprisingly, they rejected our gesture outright but warned us to be careful. What a mayhem in Southern Kaduna and what an uncommon favor bestowed on some members of NIGEP by the gallant men of the Nigerian army!

THE BESIEGE THAT HONORED PRESIDENT JIMMY CARTER!

On a long field trip, driving far into the night while visiting Local Government Areas (LGAs) endemic for Guinea worm in Niger, Kebbi and Zamfara States to collect village monthly surveillance reports, distribute filters and other interventions materials, pay field staff, and convey dozens of newly donated bicycles from Ilorin to Gusau, (Zamfara State) for use during interventions by the Village-Based Health Workers, the devil was on the road.

At about midnight, the three-man NIGEP team on the trip encountered a massive road block (unknown to them, it was mounted by a gang of armed robbers who were posing as uniformed law enforcement agents). In a twinkling of an eye, some eight unruly armed men had surrounded the vehicle to ascertain its contents and probably snatch the vehicle.

The panic-stricken staff informed the besiegers that they were members of the Guinea eradication team. One of the nasty besiegers struck the body of the pick-up van and demanded to know why the team was travelling at that odd time. Pushing the driver off, he insisted that all the filters, bicycles, drums of Abate chemical and other contents of the vehicle should be off-loaded. The salaries for the NIGEP field staff in some 40 LGAs in Sokoto, Zamfara, Katsina, and Kogi States were in a bag kept under loads of filters and bicycles. Fearing that the gang would uncover the money if the vehicle was searched, the NIGEP staff repeated that they were members of the Guinea worm eradication team. The superior commander of the gang exclaimed "OK, you are the Jimmy Carter people. He is doing good work. Leave them. Let them go"!

The NIGEP staff hurriedly and nervously drove off. About 2 km from the road block, the NIGEP team met long lines of commercial and private vehicles who were astonished how the NIGEP/The Carter Center team managed to get through the armed robbers who had besieged the road for the past several hours. That was when the NIGEP team knew that the besiegers were actually armed robbers and not policemen. The good name and work of former American President, Hon. Jimmy Carter, were honored by the gang during the horrific ordeal. Thus, through the mercy of God, the NIGEP team passed through fire unburnt and survived the flood without drowning!

THIS SLEEP WAS NOT UNTO DEATH!

A training workshop on integrated surveillance was scheduled to hold in Katsina. Dr. Henry Edeghere, a WHO Consultant, was the lead resource person. My driver and I had travelled through Niger, Kebbi, Sokoto, and Zamfara States all day, collecting monthly surveillance reports and replenishing materials for interventions. While in Minna, the driver developed severe malaria.

After receiving treatment in the hospital and resting for a while, I had to take over the driving because he was too weak and drowsy to drive. In Gusau, in the mist of acute fuel scarcity, I had to queue for more than 3 h. Unavoidably, we arrived in Katsina for the workshop very late and spent almost an hour looking for hotel accommodation because virtually all the rooms had been booked except a small one which I surrendered to the driver because of his health. I then returned to the Katsina Guest House, the venue of the workshop. With no room and in the peak of early morning hamatan, I slept in the Land Cruiser with the windows closed because of the hamatan cold.

As a back-up, two plastic jerrycans of petrol were bought in Guasu and stored in the boot of the vehicle. With my deplorable sense of smell, I slept deeply. The four doors and the boot of the Land Cruiser were locked securely from inside. In the morning, when participants had assembled for the workshop, the organizers were desperately looking for me. They saw my vehicle parked but saw neither me nor my driver, who was still sick in his hotel. At about 10.00 a.m., one of the participants moved closer and peeped into my Land Cruiser only to see me fast asleep! They shouted my name and banged on the vehicle several time with no response until Dr. Edeghere made a bigger bang on the vehicle and shouted "Prof" very loudly. I heard him faintly, as if from a long distance and responded weakly. He instructed me to unlock the door. I did and I was thus rescued and treated. I was in the jaws of death but similar to what **Jesus Christ** said of Lazarus in the **Holy Bible**, my sleep was not unto death but to eliminate dracunculiasis and its scourge and to glorify God!

CHAPTER 14

The Unsung but Remarkable Grassroots Stakeholders in Dracunculiasis Elimination in Nigeria

SOME SPECTACULAR ROLES OF CHILDREN IN DRACUNCULIASIS ELIMINATION

Case 1: A Major Disaster Averted by an 8-Year-Old Girl

Locally fabricated baft cloth materials from textile factories and markets were used initially for filters in the dracunculiasis elimination program until a more refined, lighter, more attractive and free nylon monofilament filters were donated in large quantities to the Nigeria Guinea Worm Eradication Programme (NIGEP) through The Carter Center. The distribution and use of filters was one of the core and most cost-effective intervention strategies adopted by NIGEP. Others were safe drinking water supply, vector control, using temephos (Abate) and health education.

On a particular occasion, a large consignment of fabricated nylon monofilament filters were imported. Some 2.5 million pieces were supplied to NIGEP North West Zone for an average distribution of three to five filters per household in all the endemic villages. The distribution of these new filters commenced in Tsakatsa village, Rimi LGAs, Katsina State. During the third National Case Search, the village had 604 cases of Guinea worm. There was neither a hand-dug well nor a borehole in the village. Some 30 min after the commencement of the filter distribution to households, an 8-year-old girl ran to me that her household filter was bad. We laughed and boastfully told her that it was a brand new filter imported from abroad and that it could not be bad. She confidently insisted and showed me some very tiny but visible holes that were most likely caused by the needles of the machine used for the sewing. On her particular filter, we counted up to 15 tiny holes. A member of our intervention team jokingly described each of the holes as "big enough for an elephant to pass through." Figuratively, he was referring to the ease with which cyclops could pass through the holes into the drinking water without being filtered out.

As mentioned earlier, cyclops are the mandatory intermediate host in the transmission of Guinea worm disease to man through drinking water; i.e., without cyclops, there is no dracunculiasis. In rapid succession, all the filter distributors in the village inspected and circled with markers as many filters as they could inspect. More than 500 new filters checked that day were punctured, defective and unsuitable to filter out cyclops, making the drinking water unsafe. At the zonal office, more than 2500 new filters randomly picked and checked, from different batches, were all punctured, bearing multiple tiny but visible holes caused by the manufacturer's needles during sewing. Consequently, all the new filters already distributed in the village and those distributed to all the NIGEP zones were withdrawn from being distributed.

The exceptional vigilance of this little girl had the following significance:

1. It demonstrated the efficacy and benefit of intensive and sustained health education at the user level that all filters must be carefully kept and checked at all times before being used to filter drinking water;

2. It justified the benefits of carrying the users at the grassroots along and receiving feedback from them through sustained monitoring, supervision, and evaluation;

3. It confirms that the better eyesight of children than their parents was an asset in detecting and identifying defected, torn or punctured filters that should not be used to filter pond water before consumption in villages endemic for Guinea worm disease;

4. The vigilance of the little girl helped to prevent the delay of dracunculiasis elimination in Nigeria beyond year 2013 when the World Health Organization (WHO) officially certified Nigeria free of dracunculiasis and

5. The little girl might be unsung but posterity will remember her gallant role and courage to "say incessantly something when she saw something"!

The Eradication of Dracunculiasis (Guinea Worm Disease) in Nigeria. https://doi.org/10.1016/B978-0-12-816764-9.00014-6

Case 2: The Invincible Abdullahi: The Infected 4-Year-Old Boy With the Bigger Heart of All!

I was photocopying some Guinea worm disease forms in Gusau market when a petty trader came and reported to me that there was an outbreak of dracunculiasis in Kaura Namoda. Kaura Namoda is the railway terminus in North Western Nigeria and the headquarters of Kaura Namoda Local Government Areas (LGA). The public had been extensively encouraged to make such a report. The Global 2000/The Carter Center vehicle made our identification easy.

Kaura Namoda is about 50 km from Gusau, the Zamfara State capital. Notwithstanding, a rapid response surveillance team was dispatched immediately to Kaura Namoda. At the LGA Secretariat, the outbreak was denied but it was rumored that there were some cases at the Federal Polytechnic in the town. At the Polytechnic, that weekend, some 30—40 students were gathered for any information on dracunculiasis cases in the school. They confirmed that two students were infected and that the outbreak was at Yankaba, about 5 km away. At Yankaba village and with the help of some Polytechnic students, a rapid random door-to-door case search for about 30 minutes revealed more than 50 active cases of dracunculiasis.

There were only three shallow hand-dug wells, including the one located at the dispensary in the village. The only existing borehole had broken down and had been abandoned for more than 10 years. The following day, multiple intervention teams were mobilized and dispatched to Yankaba from Gusau to launch a health education campaign, distribute filters and commence rehabilitation of the abandoned borehole. The NIGEP/The Carter Center team in the zone had the expertise to repair and maintain boreholes.

The District Head was not readily available, most members of the community were unwilling to disclose the source of their drinking ponds (so that a team could apply vector control using temephos) and the use of the dangerous, unhealthy, traditional method of managing cases of Guinea worm disease with **Sekia** was rampant. Amid these inhibitions and challenges, the zonal office considered the large-scale surgical extraction of Guinea worms as a most cost-effective intervention in the short term. The community dispensary was used as the extraction center. Several villagers gathered as spectators, but only an insignificant few came forward for extraction because of fear based on their experience with **Sekia**. The few whose Guinea worms were extracted were exclusively children who were forced by parents, relatives and teachers. Strikingly, Abdullahi, a 4-year-old boy with multiple infections on both feet, was forcefully presented for extraction. Surprisingly, he insisted that he should be allowed to sit down by himself. Two elderly men wanted to hold Abdullahi down as the extraction began but Abdullahi insisted that he should be left alone. To the bewilderment of all the onlookers (young, old, men, women and children), Abdullahi, with four emerging worms, neither cried nor resisted as the extractions proceeded. As the third extraction began, Abdullahi broke his silence for the first time. "Na gode likita" (thank you Doctor), he said. Spontaneously, everybody clapped and hailed Abdullahi in disbelief of his exceptional courage and big heart. Thereafter, older men, women and other children willingly came forward for their own extractions. Recovery was dramatic and the villagers hailed and embraced the procedure.

We could not finish the extraction exercise that day because there were so many cases with multiple infections. On arrival the following day for the remaining extractions, many more infected people than expected had gathered and were waiting for us at the dispensary. Infected victims from adjacent villages had also come forward because they had seen or heard about the extraction and the dramatic recovery that Abdullahi and others had made within 24 hours after the surgical extraction of their worms.

After three days, the abandoned borehole had been successfully rehabilitated by Engineers Saka and Joseph Omonayin, staff of the NIGEP/The Carter Center North West Zone office. We had also successfully identified and treated with temephos the pond from where the villagers were fetching their drinking water. With these interventions, dracunculiasis was rapidly eliminated in Yankaba, more than 10 years before Nigeria was certified free of dracunculiasis in 2013 by the WHO.

Case 3: The One Naira that Exposed Guinea Worm Infection for Elimination

The endemicity of dracunculiasis had repeatedly been rumored in Kubuta, Goronyo LGA, Sokoto State. However, the community had consistently denied the report. On a fateful afternoon, we were making yet another attempt to unravel the hidden endemicity of Kunkunu (Guinea worm disease) in the village. As we walked down the narrow path from the main road to the village, we met a 7 year-old girl (Hauwa) who greeted us very politely but nervously. To reward her for her impressive native manner, I gave her one naira. She received it joyfully and gratefully. That spurred me to ask her if there was any case of dracunculiasis in her village. She nodded positively and asked us to follow her. In the first household she took us to, we saw three bad cases of Guinea worm infection. Hauwa took us to five households where we counted 23 cases of dracunculiasis before some elderly men came, grabbed her, and wanted to beat her for exposing cases of the infection, which hitherto they had been hiding. Our pleading saved her from punishment. We seized the opportunity to explain our mission of assisting to eliminate the horror of the infection in the village. After discussing with the Maigari (village head), we identified 67 cases of the infection in our door-to-door case search.

Thereafter, all the dracunculiasis interventions (health education; filter distribution; vector control using temephos and surgical worm extraction) were carried out. Most delightfully, when we brought the problem to the attention of the LGA Chairman and Deputy Governor of Sokoto State (now a Senator), Alhaji Aliyu Magatakarda Wamakko, they ensured that three hand-dug wells and a solar-pumped borehole were promptly provided. These water sources were among those commissioned by Gen. Dr. Yakubu Gowon (the former Nigeria Head of State) and the Sokoto State Executives in April 2001. Two years after the interventions, dracunculiasis was permanently eliminated in the village. **What a golden one naira!**

Case 4: The Folk Song and the Elimination of Dracunculiasis in Korowa, Kwara State

A remarkable innovation in the NIGEP/The Carter Center North West Zone was the effective and sustainable public awareness mounted in all the States, LGAs and villages. Individuals and communities were empowered to report any case of dracunculiasis seen and to apply all the preliminary interventions immediately (e.g., prevent the infected person(s) from entering and contaminating the community source(s) of drinking ponds and to report cases immediately).

Compliance with the application of this innovation was impressively demonstrated by the Korowa community in the Ilorin East LGA of Kwara State. This was the last endemic community in Kwara State. The outbreak occurred after dracunculiasis was considered eliminated in the State. The Korowa community alleged that an infected animal breeder from a northern State had contaminated their pond. They also alleged that when the outbreak was reported to the Local Government Chief Executive, he declined to assist because the community did not vote for him in the election that the Chief Executive eventually won.

Remaining undaunted, the community took their destiny into their own hands by applying the preliminary interventions as had been imparted to them. They set up a pond guard and banned any infected

person from entering their pond. They wrote down the names and gender of the 23 infected victims and took a group photograph. Within 48 hours, they had taken this evidence to the State Epidemiological Unit in Ilorin, to UNICEF-assisted Ruwatsan in Ilorin, and to NIGEP/The Global 2000 North West Zone Office in Ilorin. The delegates to the three offices were led in folk song by a 10-year-old female composer and singer of the Guinea worm song.

An urgent meeting of officials of the three agencies that the community delegates had visited was held. The specific roles of the epidemiology unit, UNICEF-Ruwatsan and NIGEP/Global 2000 to manage the outbreak were identified. By 8.00 a.m. the following day, Mr. Adegboye, the UNICEF-Ruwatsan Project Manager had mobilized two drilling rigs to the community, about 30 km away. Amid drumming and folk songs, borehole drilling began at two sites. Health education was intensified. Filters were distributed to all persons who were 8 years and above in the community. The community was also mobilized and empowered to construct a Ventilated Improved Pit (VIP) latrine. Five days later, the two boreholes and three VIP latrines had been completed and commissioned amid celebrations, feasting, drumming, and dancing to the beautiful songs led by Fatima, the 10-year-old girl.

E ma se a dupe

(Thank you, we are grateful)

E fun wa l'omi tuntun

(You gave us new water)

Aiye nyin na yio si tuntun

(Your life shall be new)

No case of dracunculiasis was recorded a year later! About 10 years after the outbreak and as a pre-certification requirement by WHO, my team re-visited Korowa village in 2009. The seven-man evaluation team arrived in the village at about 8.30 p.m. Surprisingly, despite of the night darkness and using only a hurricane lamp, after introducing our mission, two of the younger men spontaneously recognized Dr. Edungbola, even by name. Fatima, the 10-year-old singer of folk songs had married and had twins. The boys and girls who were 10 years old or younger and who had gathered to see the "night visitors," did not know what a Guinea worm is! Dracunculiasis had gone forever in the Korowa community! Agricultural, educational, economic, health, socio-cultural and religious activities were boosted at a magnitude unprecedented in the history of the community.

THE SPECTACULAR ROLE OF WOMEN IN DRACUNCULIASIS ELIMINATION

A substantial number of married women in the NIGEP North West Zone faithfully observe their religious injunctions of being in *Purdah*. Strikingly, that did not inhibit them in their distinct roles in the elimination of dracunculiasis in their respective communities. The general role played by women in the elimination of Guinea worm disease included filtration of pond water before storing and making it available for family consumption; the possession, use, maintenance and replacement of damaged filters and the banning of infected victims from entering and contaminating the community drinking ponds. An example of a special role played by women in dracunculiasis elimination in the zone is presented below.

The Revolt That Accelerated the Elimination of Dracunculiasis in an Endemic Community

Dutse-Wake was notorious as a leading community endemic for Guinea worm in Birnin Magaji LGA, Zamfara State. Surgical Guinea worm extraction and comprehensive case management had become an exceptionally rapid, acceptable and cost-effective intervention that brought dramatic relief and recovery for the victims. It also drastically reduced the risk of water contamination and the spread of the disease.

An unusually large number of Guinea worm cases (many with multiple infections and severe complications) had occurred in Dutse-Wake. Hence, the surgical extraction team, under the leadership of Solomon Olukade, was mobilized to the village for interventions. The first 2 days of extraction were remarkably successful as 98 cases were comprehensively managed. Among the cases managed was that of a middle-aged man with five emerging worms and severe complications. He had been incapacitated and bedridden for more than 3 weeks. The following day, after the successful extraction of his worms and comprehensive management of his wounds, he was the first person in his household to wake up for the morning prayer. His three wives and other members of his household were astonished by his sudden wellness. The three wives who were also infected were wondering what their husband had used to bring him that dramatic recovery. Hitherto, the women in the community had been deceived by the men that the Guinea worm extraction team were collecting blood and taking it to Lagos. When the wives pressed their husband harder on what he had used and demanded that he should give them the same, the husband disclosed the source of his recovery. Very rapidly, the information had spread to other women in the

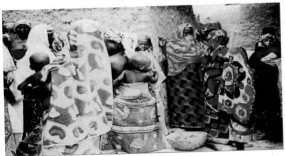

FIG. 14.1 Protest by women that husbands were deceiving them and stopping them from benefiting from surgical extraction of Guinea worms.

community. The women revolted, refusing to cook and perform other essential domestic responsibilities (Fig. 14.1). The matter was brought to the attention of the NIGEP North West Zone office in Gusau. A compromise was reached whereby infected women would first be attended to at an enclosed compound specified by the men. Thereafter, the men would take their turns in the open central market (under the shade of a big Dogonyaro tree) which was easily accessible to all the victims in that community. The arrangement worked out very successfully. A similar arrangement was adopted in most other socio-culturally and religiously similar communities. The accrued benefit therefrom was the accelerated elimination of dracunculiasis in those communities and in the zone in general. It was most gratifying that the women accepted the men's apology. Thus, there was no permanent animosity but domestic harmony!

REMARKABLE ROLES OF ELEMENTARY SCHOOLS IN DRACUNCULIASIS ELIMINATION

As a frontline beneficiary and stakeholder, on a short- and long-term basis, elementary school children played a very significant and crucial role in the elimination of dracunculiasis in the NIGEP North West Zone.

In particular, their role included rapid case detection and reporting, quality control of surveillance activities and the household distribution and usage of filters, especially in relatively large endemic communities and in circumstances when the endemic community was inaccessible from outside because of floods.

With the assistance and full cooperation of primary school teachers, intensive school-based health education on the transmission, impact, prevention and benefits of the elimination of dracunculiasis was mounted and replicated. Children were initially mobilized and motivated, using audio-visuals, coloring books, game books, crayons, pencils, posters and surveillance booklets in Ajamin (i.e., surveillance booklets in Hausa language but written in Arabic).

Every morning on school days, each class teacher took and recorded the attendance register. In addition, he/she asked each pupil if there was any new case of dracunculiasis in his/her household (provide names and gender, if yes). The teacher also enquired if the pupil saw or knew of any new case of dracunculiasis in the community. Any positive response was compared and harmonized with the report in the Village Based Health Worker's (VBHW) surveillance book. On weekends, Sundays and during public holidays, pupils were encouraged to report to the teachers, VBHWs and/or NIGEP/LGA Guinea worm staff in the locality. Various incentives (coloring books, crayons, pencils, etc.) and sometimes transport money (if it involved travelling to the LGA headquarters or State Capital to report outbreaks) were provided to encourage effective participation and reporting.

At the onset, as part of the school-based interventions, every pupil by household was given the number of filters that corresponded to the number of persons (8 years and older) in the household. Thus, every eligible member of the household possessed at least one filter. The pupils also ensured the regular and correct use of the filters in the household, the good condition of filters and the replacement of worn out or damaged filters. Because the school children played a major role in the household fetching water, they also played an additional role in preventing infected persons from entering and contaminating community drinking ponds and reporting immediately when such contamination occurred so that it could be treated promptly with temephos for vector control.

The school children also provided useful information on traditional practitioners in the community who were using **Sekia** secretly and, thereby, inflicting avoidable complications of Guinea worm infection, which could be fatal or lead to irreversible deformities among the victims. As an important practical component of school-based interventions, every class had a UNICEF-WATSAN pot with a tap. The class prefect and teacher ensured that pond water was properly filtered before storage for consumption in the school. The elementary school-based intervention strategy for dracunculiasis elimination was cost-effective, reliable and sustainable, especially in large communities. What an unsung but very commendable role of the elementary school children in dracunculiasis elimination!

AGED AND RETIRED BUT STILL CONTRIBUTING REMARKABLY TO DRACUNCULIASIS ELIMINATION

Activities and conditions involved in dracunculiasis elimination are unimaginably tasking, rigorous, demanding and called for uncommon sacrifices, especially for those aged 70 years or more. In the NIGEP North West Zone, circumstances were even more challenging and excruciating for retired elderly persons because the exercise involved travelling hundreds of kilometers away from home and family; covering six vast States with several LGAs and many hard-to-reach rural communities during the heavy rainy season, which coincided with the peak of transmission, leaving the field base as early as 7:00 a.m. and returning as late as 9:00 p.m., with no food and no water all day; risking exposure to infections, zoonotic diseases, and fatigue and working whole heartedly among helpless, disadvantaged, dracunculiasis impoverished, and incapacitated villagers where conditions were pathetically complicated by malnutrition, concomitant infections, ignorance, and poverty.

Those were the conditions under which two of my aged teachers and my elder brother, in their retirements, made personal sacrifices to accelerate the elimination of Guinea worm disease in the NIGEP North West Zone. Gen. Dr. Yakubu Gowon, Nigeria's former Head of State, was also an epitome of such sacrifices as he incessantly promoted advocacy and community mobilization for the elimination of dracunculiasis and its adverse impoverishment in Nigeria.

In order to utilize the resources and logistic support provided by The Carter Center for dracunculiasis elimination in the NIGEP North West Zone to the maximum and based on our collective determination to accelerate the elimination of the disease in the zone, I sought and obtained the willingness of two of my old teachers and my elder brother (with relevant expertise) to help bridge some technical gaps and lapses in our field operations. Despite being retired and elderly professionals in their respective career specializations, they willingly accepted to help in the following core intervention strategies: surgical Guinea worm extraction and comprehensive case management; vector control using temephos; refined high-level advocacy and community mobilization; training/re-training and motivation of The Carter Center Field Staff; the promotion of sustainable health education and the implementation of effective monitoring and evaluation of field activities. The elimination of dracunculiasis, especially in the highly endemic communities (such as Turtsawa, Garin Serkin Adar, Nassarawa Mailayi, Karadua, Tungan Gana,

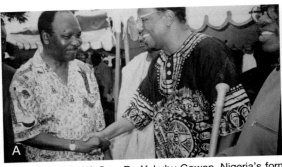
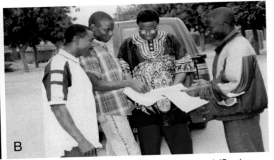

FIG. 14.2 **(A)** Gen. Dr. Yakubu Gowon, Nigeria's former Head of State and Dr. Job. O. Adewunmi (Senior NIGEP Consultant and a retired top education administrator) sharing a warm handshake during advocacy and intervention activities in the NIGEP North West Zone. **(B)** Dr. Job O. Adewunmi (center), Senior Consultant, NIGEP/The Carter Center North West Zone is seen with four Senior Zone Field Managers (left to right: A.A. Sanyaolu; Engr. Saka; Dr. Job O. Adewunmi, and Moses Atolagbe) discussing critical intervention issues to accelerate the elimination of Guinea worm disease in the LGAs.

Gusami, Yankaba, Modomawa, Tidi Bali, Leka, Ajenejo, Olubojo, Kubuta, Kaikazaka I and II, Turame, Tsogawa, Tsakatsa Sango, Hayin Samawa, etc.) could have been much delayed without the reinforcements provided by the retired trio.

Below are brief notes as a tribute to the three unsung retired civil servants who quietly made exceptional sacrifices that fast tracked the elimination of dracunculiasis in the NIGEP North West Zone

1. **Pa Elder J.A. Omidiji:**

   He was my class teacher in 1956 (about 60 years ago) when I was in Junior Primary Two. He had considerable experience working with physically challenged persons in Ibadan for years. He eventually retired as the Chief Community Mobilization Officer for UNICEF/RUWATSAN in Kwara/Kogi State. He used his past connections effectively in the aforementioned endemic States to strengthen advocacy, community mobilization and health education.

2. **Elder Dr. J.A. Adewunmi:** (Fig. 14.2A and B)

   He was my secondary school and Higher School Certificate teacher in 1963, 1964 and 1968. He was a most celebrated secondary school principal in Kwara/Kogi State, having won best results award in WASCE for three consecutive years. He was an authority in chemistry, the experience he applied for effective treatment of hundreds of drinking ponds with temephos. This was a very cost-effective vector control strategy in dracunculiasis elimination. He also trained and supervised many field staff in the application of temephos. Dr. Adewunmi also played a major role in advocacy, community mobilization, and the motivation of all field staff. He retired

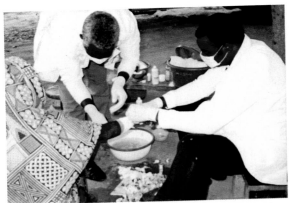

FIG. 14.3 Pa. Edungbola, a retired Director in the Ministry of Health (left) and Olukade, Senior Medical Staff in the NIGEP North West Zone (right) surgically extracting and managing three emerging adult female Guinea worms on the body of a housewife.

voluntarily as a lecturer at the University of Ilorin. He was the Chairman of the Teaching Service Commission in Kwara and Kogi States. Amid all the challenges, Dr. Adewunmi played a remarkable role in the timely elimination of a stunning outbreak of dracunculiasis in the Dekina LGAs of Kogi State (his home State).

3. **Pa. Elder E.A. Edungbola:**

   He retired in 1995 as Director of Nursing in the Kwara State Ministry of Health. He was endowed with rich experience in the nursing profession, having worked in Government Hospitals in Kaduna, Kano, Birnin Kudu, Lokoja and Ilorin. He also

Consultant. This insinuation was probably based on speculated or falsely rumored blackmail and an attempt by the management to confirm the erroneous allegation.

I was never personally disturbed, being strengthened by the Biblical urge to be steadfast, immovable and abundant in good works. Besides, I believe that "all things are naked and open to the eyes of Him to whom we must all give account." With those convictions, all staff of the NIGEP North West Zone, under the example of my leadership, continued to labor with absolute dedication to achieve the levels of performance that were faultless, exemplary and exceptional in Nigeria.

Despite a most extensive coverage area in nine highly endemic States (Federal Capital Territory, Abuja, Kaduna, Katsina, Kebbi, Kogi, Kwara, Niger, Sokoto, and Zamfara), I visited all my endemic States, LGAs and villages most regularly, most religiously and most cost-effectively with unmatched holistic interventions (including several potent radical innovations), which were executed by the best and most disciplined field staff. Also, my zonal advocacy campaigns and community participation were unparalleled and sustainable. In addition, I knew all my LGAs and villages by name and could drive to all my endemic LGAs and villages, unguided. I was well known in all the endemic LGAs and villages.

By coincidence, that very week when the sugar-cane seller testified by his unguided and uninfluenced conscience (as on the previous three occasions when similar identity questions were asked), the NIGEP/The Carter Center team visited the government office in Sokoto, the State Capital. Alh. Aliyu Magatakarada Wamakko, the Deputy Governor and the only Deputy Governor who was also the Chairman of the State Guinea Worm Taskforce in Nigeria, received us warmly and commended the NIGEP/The Carter Center staff for the excellent work being carried out. In his remarks, he added that "Yes, for the Professor, Guinea worm eradication is not just his passion but his life, his ID, his nationality and his religion." That was a sufficient and personal joy, second only to the elimination of dracunculiasis itself!

Thereafter, dracunculiasis was speedily eliminated in the three remaining endemic LGAs (Sabon Birnin, Goroyo and Isa) in Sokoto State. What a blessing and reward for a most active commitment to dracunculiasis elimination! Alhaji Wammako became the Executive Governor of Sokoto State (for two terms). Currently, he is an Honorable Senator in the Upper House in Abuja.

My commitment and passion for dracunculiasis elimination in Nigeria as a cause of an unnecessary suffering and suffering from an unnecessary cause was natural, being motivated by my earliest encounters with the disease as mentioned in Chapter 3. As early as 1978, my University research team had initiated extensive epidemiological mapping, advocacy, community mobilization and health education against dracunculiasis. Thereafter, UNICEF, The Carter Center, WHO, the United Nations Development Programme, the Federal Government of Nigeria, the Yakubu Gowon Centre and other stakeholders became indispensable catalysts by providing all the necessary resources, encouragement and enablement for the elimination of dracunculiasis in Nigeria. The encouragement of UNICEF at the outset and the consistency of the support of The Carter Center throughout the elimination drive, were most remarkable and unquestionably decisive.

Today, I have learnt, remained satisfied and been consoled that the integrity of a man is what he does when no one is watching. Besides, "God is not unjust to forget our good work and labor."

In the case of the sugar-cane seller at Garin Serkin Adar, there was no mistaking my identity. However, I had experienced mistaken identity before. On an occasion, one Chief Eba, from an LGA hyperendemic for dracunculiasis in Benue State, had come, wanting to see me in the office. After being invited to please sit down, he requested to see Professor Edungbola. "Yes, I am" was my answer. He responded objectionably that he wanted to see the Professor and not his Personal Assistant. I repeated that "I am he." Chief Eba sounded very disgusted, declaring that he was disappointed because he was expecting to see a very tall and old man with gray hair and a wrinkled face. Praise God, at that time, I had been a Professor at the University of Ilorin for more than a decade.

"Do you know him?" is better than "do you know who I am?" For if you have to tell people who you are, you probably really are not who you think you are!

AN UNCOMMON PRIVILEGE DURING THE DRACUNCULIASIS ELIMINATION CAMPAIGN

General Dr. Yakubu Gowon (retired), the former Head of State and the incumbent Chairman of the Yakubu Gowon Centre, is an exceptional and a most remarkable Nigerian with intimidating historical antecedents. He was the youngest and the longest serving Head of State Nigeria has ever produced. During his tenure as Nigeria's Head of State, both the Organisation of African Unity and the Economic Community of West African States were established, the National Youth Service

Corps (NYSC) was launched, the Nigeria's civil war was fought and won with unconditional reconciliation and the Kainji Dam was impounded to generate hydroelectric power for national consumption (among many other achievements during his tenure). To date, Gen. Yakubu Gowon remains the only Nigerian Head of State with an academic PhD. Despite these and many other attributes, Gen. Dr. Gowon remains most humble, amiable, approachable, accessible, godly, prayerful, patriotic, most respected and most admired. Anyone would want to associate with Gen. Dr. Gowon for the awesomeness of his life and character.

With an uncommon humility, patriotism, and relentless services to Nigeria in various capacities, Gen. Dr. Gowon gladly accepted the invitation by the former American President, Hon. Jimmy Carter and his wife, Rosalynn Carter (Chairman of The Carter Center, Atlanta GA, USA) to help strengthen advocacy for dracunculiasis elimination in Nigeria at a very critical time when the elimination of the disease seemed to be experiencing a form of stagnation and it was almost certain that the 1995 target deadline could not be met.

As scheduled by Dr. E.S. Miri, the first Nigerian to be The Carter Center Country Representative, Gen. Dr. Gowon had arrived on an advocacy visit to Zamfara State, the most endemic State in the NIGEP North West Zone where I was the NIGEP/The Carter Center Senior Zonal Consultant. Together with some senior members of my zonal staff, we went to welcome the former Head of State in the office of the Deputy Governor of Zamfara State. The retired General was indescribably simple, humorous, kind and always had something remarkable to say to or about everybody present. It was laughter galore. Everyone felt free, recognized, happy and motivated.

There and then, as we were arranging the logistics of going to Birnin Magaji, the most Guinea worm hyperendemic LGA in Zamfara State, the unexpected happened. The uncommon privilege and recognition unfolded when our former Head of State announced that I should be riding with him in his vehicle and insisted that I should be sitting by his side! I was most nervous and uncomfortable as we drove through the rough make-shift road for about 2 h. The retired General asked me many technical questions on Guinea worms and Guinea worm disease, its history, its complications and its implications, including the magnitude of the resulting impoverishment in endemic communities.

I was humbled when the retired General and an academic PhD holder told me he had been reading several reports on dracunculiasis in Nigeria and that he enjoyed and understood my zonal reports best. He explained that he wanted to know more about the disease so that he could serve and help most effectively. As nervous and humbled as I was, I narrated several heart-wrenching experiences and encounters with dracunculiasis to him.

When I was sufficiently relaxed, I told His Excellency how I took a photograph of his framed portrait in my principal's office at Titcombe College (when he became the Head of State) and made good sales and profits from many black and white prints I sold to students. The General jokingly demanded his own royalties. General Dr. Yakubu Gowon's advocacy role was timely, effective and rewarding.

The late President Musa Yaardua (when he was the Executive Governor of Katsina State), the late Prince Audu Abubarkar (the Executive Governor of Kogi State) and Alh. Attahiru D. Bafarawa (the Executive Governor of Sokoto State) with his Deputy Governor (Senator Aliyu Magatakarda Wamakko), among others, took full advantage of General Gowon's advocacy campaigns and eliminated endemic dracunculiasis in their respective States in record time.

CHAPTER 16

Blessings of Some Uncommon Circumstances Encountered During Dracunculiasis Elimination in Nigeria

THE COMMANDANT'S FAVORABLE DISCRETION WHEN IT REALLY MATTERED

Priority activities at the onset of dracunculiasis elimination in Nigeria were the establishment of national committees, the inauguration of State Task Forces and the printing and dispatching of forms for training, case searching and soft interventions. Dates for trainings and field activities had been scheduled. Forms were printed centrally in Lagos but arrived only 2 days before the commencement of training and field activities in the North West Zone. I had arranged with my official driver that we would be leaving Ilorin by 5.00 a.m. to deliver the forms to all the States in the Nigeria Guinea Worm Eradication Programme (NIGEP) North West Zone: Niger; Sokoto (currently Sokoto, Kebbi, and Zamfara States); Katsina; Federal Capital Territory, Abuja; Kwara (now Kwara and Kogi States) and Kaduna.

On arriving at the driver's residence the following morning as scheduled, I discovered he was indisposed and could not travel. I had no option but to set out alone. The first delivery of the forms was at Minna, Niger State. Thereafter, I travelled and delivered forms to Sokoto, Katsina, Federal Capital Territory and Kaduna States that same day! I arrived and slept at Dubar Hotel Kaduna at about 11.00 p.m. As I was to preside over the Kwara State Guinea Worm Taskforce Meeting the following day in Ilorin at 11.00 a.m., I left the hotel very early, arriving at the toll gate near the airport at about 4.00 a.m. I was shocked and disappointed when I arrived at the toll gate only to meet long queues of assorted vehicles blocking everyone. There was a standing official security rule against entering Kaduna before 6.00 a.m.

Pressed by the urgency to preside over a crucial Guinea worm disease meeting in Ilorin at 11.00 a.m. and despite what looked like a futile exercise, I summoned the courage to approach the military commandant, introduced myself and informed him of my mission and its importance. Surprisingly, almost immediately, the commandant personally commenced the clearing of trailers, heavy trucks, commercial buses and all vehicles blocking the highway. After about 30 min, I was exclusively led through the multitude of vehicles blocking the highway. Just before 11.00 a.m., I arrived in Ilorin and presided over the meeting. Members of the Task Force were astonished that I had made such a marathon journey within 24 h.

What an uncommon favor! It was a most appreciated and significant gesture toward successfully launching of dracunculiasis eradication activities in the NIGEP North West Zone!

A CHALLENGING BEGINNING THAT ACCELERATED DRACUNCULIASIS ELIMINATION IN ZAMFARA STATE

When the late General Sanni Abacha created Zamfara and Kebbi States out of the old Sokoto State, one of the natural liabilities shared by the trio was 20%, 30% and 50% dracunculiasis endemicity in Sokoto, Kebbi and Zamfara States, respectively. A rapid active Guinea worm case search by the NIGEP North West Zone team revealed an alarming hyperendemicity of Guinea worm disease in the Local Government Areas (LGAs) of Birmin Magaji, Bukkuyum, Bungudu, Anka, Tsafe and Kaura Namoda in the new Zamfara State. At that time, of the four NIGEP core intervention strategies in the zone (safe water supply, vector control using temephos [Abate], filter distribution and health education), only health education was a readily available and feasible option.

An alternative and very promising radical innovation was large-scale surgical extraction of Guinea worms. The constraint against this strategy was lack of materials for worm extraction and wound management (antiseptics, antibiotics, analgesics, bandages, xylocaine solution, bivalcin sprays, surgical blades, forceps, hand gloves, etc.).

When the State Director General of Health (Alh. Suleiman Bello) was briefed on the prospects and constraints of the worm extraction strategy, he personally visited some hyperendemic communities to see the magnitude of the problem himself. After seeing what he described as "horribly pathetic," he advised that a cost estimate of materials needed should be urgently provided. When that was promptly done, he was highly impressed that the financial request made was far less than his minimum expectation of the amount that would be needed to effectively manage the alarming number of cases in all the hyperendemic villages and LGAs in the State. When the Director General took the request to the Military Governor of the newly created Zamfara State (Col. Bala Yakubu), the Governor approved the release of the funds immediately.

The commitment, approval and timely release of funds for worm extraction and wound management produced multiple benefits, including:

1. Rapid recovery of Guinea worm victims from protracted incapacitation and timely return to their farming activities at the peak of the agricultural season;
2. Prevention of severe morbidity, irreversible complications and avoidable deaths;
3. Dramatic reduction in the number of Guinea worm cases State-wide and in the number of man days lost, which prolonged incapacitation would have caused;
4. Accelerated elimination of Guinea worm disease in the newly created disadvantaged State;
5. Replication of the Guinea worm extraction strategy advantageously in the NIGEP North West Zone and in the other zones and
6. The popularity and acceptance of the strategy by State and LGA authorities and by the traditional rulers and their grassroots subjects.

At the onset of interventions, dracunculiasis elimination activities in Zamfara State were exceptionally challenging because of:

1. The widespread hyperendemicity of the disease in the new State;
2. Multiple impediments associated with human factors;
3. Inaccessibility of several hyperendemic villages and LGAs during the rainy season, which coincided with the peak of the disease transmission and
4. Lack of roads, safe water sources, rural network communications and other basic infrastructures and amenities.

It is most gratifying that the timely commitment and support of the State Government, coupled with the logistical and technical support provided by NIGEP/The

Carter Center North West Zone, averted indefinite lingering of Guinea worm disease and its adverse consequences on health, agriculture, education, demography and rapid socio-economic development in the new State.

AN UNEXPECTED REWARD FOR OUTSTANDING PERFORMANCE IN DRACUNCULIASIS ERADICATION

Group Captain Ibrahim Alkali (the Military Governor of Kwara State in 1988) played an active role in the implementation of dracunculiasis interventions in Kwara State. He was strongly influenced and supported by Dr. Abdulkarim Ibrahim (the Hon. Commissioner for Health), Alh. Kamaldeen (the Director General, Health) and Dr. J.R. Idowu (the Director, Public Health/Epidemiology Unit). Nigeria Television Authority Ilorin and the Herald newspaper were great assets (Fig. 16.1A and B).

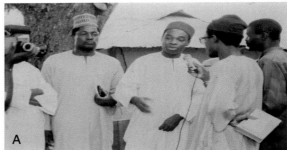

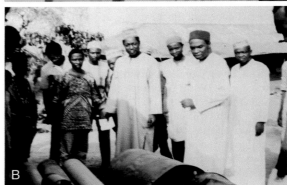

FIG. 16.1 **(A)** Kwara State Commissioner for Health, Dr. Abdulkarim Ibrahim, is exchanging views with journalists on the status of Guinea worm disease elimination in the State. Alh. Olawiyo Kamaldeen (Director General for Health) is seen on the right of the commissioner. **(B)** The Hon. Commissioner for Health with Alh. Kamaldeen (Director General for Health) and some staff of the UNICEF/WATSAN unit are seen in an endemic village with materials for sinking boreholes.

After the inauguration of the first State Guinea Worm Task Force in Anambra State, Nigeria, in 1986, under the influence of Professor A.B.C. Nwosu who was the State Hon. Commissioner for Health, Group Captain Alkali of Kwara State was among the next set of Military Governors to inaugurate State Guinea Worm Task Forces. The State Executive, under Governor Alkali, held a goodwill reception for Dr. Donald R. Hopkins and Mr. Craig Withers Jr. who led a team of Global 2000 visitors to Kwara State in July, 1988. The reception took place after the visitors had visited the University of Ilorin, Nigeria Television Authority Ilorin, and several dracunculiasis endemic villages, including Budo Ayan. Group Captain Alkali was the only Military Governor who attended the International Donors Conference at the Lagos Sheraton in 1989 to raise funds and awareness for dracunculiasis eradication.

The Nigerian President (Gen. Ibrahim Badamosi Babangida), the former USA President (Hon. Jimmy Carter and his wife, Rosalynn Carter), the late Professor Olikoye Ransome-Kuti (Hon. Minister of Health), the United Nations Development Programme (UNDP) regional director (Pierra-Claver Dambia) and His Eminence, the Sultan of Sokoto (Alh. Dr. Ibrahim Dasuki) were also present at the International Donors' Conference in 1989 (Fig. 16.2).

When Colonel Alwali Jauji Kazir was appointed to take over from Group Captain Alkali as the Military Governor of Kwara State, sustainability of the ongoing momentum for dracunculiasis elimination in the State was a concern. Hence, the State Guinea Worm Task Force, in collaboration with existing members of the State Executive, the Ministry of Health and the Directorate of Food Roads and Rural Infrastructure agreed that before the departure of the new Military Governor from Lagos to Ilorin, an arrangement would be made for him to visit the UNICEF office in Lagos. This was to sustain and strengthen the UNICEF/WATSAN activities in Kwara State with special emphasis on rural safe water supply to eliminate endemic dracunculiasis (Fig. 16.3).

After his successful visit to the UNICEF Country Representative in Lagos, Col. Alwali Kazir left Lagos for Ilorin by road. However, at Otte, Asa LGA, about 20 km from the State Capital, the new governor was persuaded to branch off at Budo-Ilorin (about 3 km from the main road), to see the Guinea worm problem and the ongoing worm extraction as arranged by the Kwara State Guinea Worm Task Force. In the village, surgical extraction of Guinea worms and case management were being led by Solomon Olukade (of the Kwara State Ministry of Health) and a member of the State Task Force.

The horrors of Guinea worm infection and the extraction and management procedures that were going

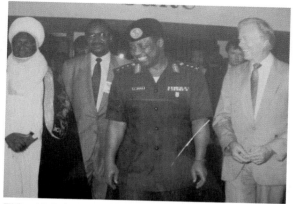

FIG. 16.2 Left to right: Alh. Dr. Ibrahim Dasuki (His Eminence, the Sultan of Sokoto); Pierra-Claver Dambia (UNDP Regional Director); President Ibrahim Babangida (former President of Nigeria) and President Jimmy Carter (the 39th American President) during the Donors' Conference at Lagos Sheraton, in 1989.

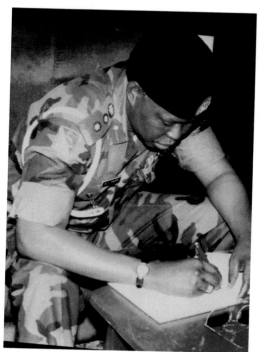

FIG. 16.3 Col. Alwali Jauji Kazir, the newly posted Military Governor to Kwara State to replace Group Captain Ibrahim Alkali, is signing the visitors' book at the UNICEF Lagos Office before the new Governor proceeded to Kwara State.

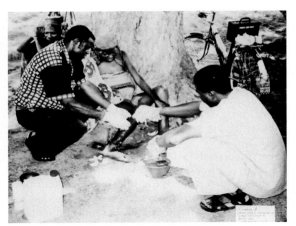

FIG. 16.4 S. Olukade (left) extracting Guinea worms from the body of a housewife. Sixty-two Guinea worms were extracted from her body during that transmission year. On the right is A. Sanyaolu, a regular assistant to Olukade for more than a decade. The victim's husband (incidentally a new Village-Based Health Worker [VBHW]) is seen behind Olukade, fearfully looking away from the extraction procedure. To the right of Sanyaolu is the VBHW's bicycle and GWD First Aid Box on the bicycle.

on overwhelmed the new Military Governor. He was so impressed by Olukade's expertise in worm extraction that he directed that Olukade should be given automatic promotion to Grade Level 11 as a reward for his dedication and commitment. In addition, the Governor directed that two boreholes (with hand pumps) should be sunk in the village from the package he negotiated with UNICEF just before he left Lagos. Thereafter, dracunculiasis was rapidly eliminated in the village within 2 years.

The unexpected promotion motivated Solomon Olukade so strongly that for more than two decades thereafter, he remained the exclusive Nigerian with exceptional proficiency and giftedness for large-scale Guinea worm extraction and comprehensive case management (Fig. 16.4). Guinea worm extraction was a unique strategy in the NIGEP North West Zone. It was very cost-effective and rapid in reducing morbidity and in accelerating the elimination of the disease in the NIGEP/The Carter Center North West Zone and in other zones.

CHAPTER 17

The Gains and Benefits of Dracunculiasis Elimination in Nigeria

In 2013, the World Health Organization (WHO) certified the Federal Republic of Nigeria free of dracunculiasis (Guinea worm disease) following the interruption of the transmission of the disease for more than three consecutive years and upon the unanimous recommendation of the International Certification Commission of Experts established by the WHO.

Nigeria's incredible achievement stunned the skeptics who had speculated at the onset of launching the eradication campaign, that Nigeria, with the highest number of infected persons globally (about 700,000 cases in some 6000 endemic villages), would be the last country to eliminate her burden of Guinea worm disease.

Thanks to the late Professor Olikoye Ransome-Kuti (Nigeria's indefatigable Honorable Minister of Health) with the full support of President Ibrahim Babangida: the United Nations Children's Fund (under the leadership of Mr. Richard Reid and his able Senior Program Officer, Mr. David Bassiouni); The Carter Center (under the Chairmanship of President Jimmy Carter and his wife, Mrs. Rosalynn Carter); the WHO (under Dr. Brew Graves, the Country Representative in Nigeria); the United Nations Development Programme.; the Japan International Cooperation Agency; Dr. Donald R. Hopkins of The Carter Center; The Carter Center Resident Advisers in Nigeria and several other groups and individuals.

As envisaged, the elimination of dracunculiasis in all endemic States (including the Federal Capital Territory, Abuja), Local Government Areas (LGAs) and communities in Nigeria has brought considerable relief, gains and benefits (Fig. 17.1A–C).

Although the post-elimination impact assessment has not been fully documented quantitatively and the benefits and gains accruing from the elimination of this ancient tormenting and impoverishing disease could be perceived differently and from different perspectives, the indisputable benefits of dracunculiasis elimination in Nigeria can be summarized as described below.

- Guinea worm disease affected virtually all facets of human life in Nigeria. Thus, the benefits accruing from the elimination of the disease have spread across agricultural, health, educational, socioeconomic, demographic, political, security, developmental and religious concerns.

  Therefore, if quantitative impact assessments are conducted, the magnitude of the gains and benefits derivable from the successful elimination of dracunculiasis in Nigeria (after so many years of its tormenting endemicity) will be astonishingly considerable.

- As a further component of health benefits, the positive impact of dracunculiasis elimination on the reduction of water-borne, water-associated, water-washed and water-related diseases is staggering. However, since these are dynamic events, sustainability and expansion of political will and action, public compliance and the continued support and cooperation of international partners and donors will be necessary to make the recorded impact an enduring gain.

- Previously infested water bodies where active transmissions were occurring every year, including ponds, broken or incomplete dams, earth dams and other stagnant surface water bodies are convertible to multiple purposes, including: irrigation for agricultural undertakings; vegetable gardening; fish ponds; animal drinking sources; clay-pot making; block fabrication, etc.

- During the early days of the search for Guinea worm cases, especially in the most recently created States and LGAs, several villages that were previously unknown at the State and LGA levels were identified and exposed for the first time.

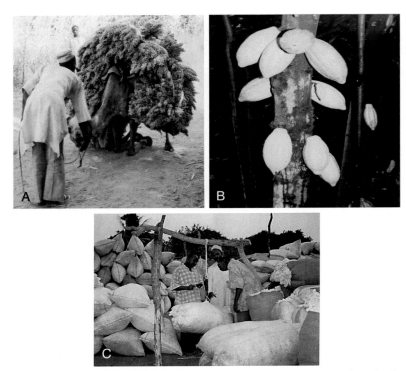

FIG. 17.1 The elimination of endemic dracunculiasis has led to more intensive and productive agricultural activities and to bumper harvests of both food **(A)** and cash crops **(B)**. **(C)** Harvested farm goods being weighed before sales.

These villages were located at the "end of the road" in the most remote and rural areas with no access roads, no schools, no safe water sources and no health facilities. In one such settlement, on seeing our vehicle emerging through the bush and sandy river beds, the villagers ran away from the village. After about 2 hours when we finally got three men (including the village head) to speak to us, they informed us that they were running away because they thought we were spirits or witches as no vehicle ever came to them before and we were the "first government people" to visit their village.

Following the discovery of such settlements and their documentation on our Guinea worm maps, the existence of such villages was brought to the attention of the LGA and State authorities. Col. Bala Yakubu, the first Military Governor of Zamfara State, played an outstanding role by creating access roads, establishing schools, constructing health facilities, and providing safe water sources to such communities. But for the elimination of dracunculiasis activities, many of those settlements would have remained unidentified, endemic, and undeveloped.

- Lessons, experiences, structures and partnerships derived from activities and events which cumulated in the dramatic elimination of dracunculiasis in Nigeria could and should be considered, modified as necessary and adopted for the implementation of other beneficial programs.
- Experiences gained through dracunculiasis elimination activities in manpower development, capacity building, skill acquisition, leadership responsibilities, resources mobilization and management and inter-partnership cooperation should be embraced, strengthened, replicated and used advantageously for the planning and implementation of control/eradication of other tropical diseases.
- Dracunculiasis elimination has led to useful and sustainable innovations, including: the advent and large-scale expansion of reasonably cheap bottled and satcheted water; the drilling of boreholes; the sinking of hand-dug wells and the construction of dams by governments, donors, communities and private individuals.

- Dracunculiasis elimination in Nigeria is a lesson that impressively demonstrates the attitudinal philosophy of not just doing what is right and worth doing but doing it well and in timely fashion!

If the elimination of Guinea worm disease in Nigeria had been delayed for just a little while longer, the unfortunate emergence, escalation and expansion of insecurities, insurgences, banditry, the magnitude of internally displaced persons, large-scale corruption, threatening lawlessness and the advent of economic recession, would have adversely prolonged the elimination of the disease indefinitely, thereby making Nigeria the last country in the world to eliminate the burdens of dracunculiasis as initially insinuated by the skeptics.

- If the successful elimination of dracunculiasis had been delayed just a bit longer, the program would have been challenged by distractions and setbacks, with potential serious conflict and competition for priority, resources, and political will against more deadly diseases, newly emerging diseases, re-emerging diseases and stagnated diseases, including Ebola virus disease; Lassa fever; HIV/AIDS; tuberculosis; malaria; malnutrition and other neglected tropical diseases.
- A most striking but unsung gain of dracunculiasis elimination in Nigeria is the "re-birth" of a new nation without the persistent, incessant, horrifying, intimidating, dehumanizing, impoverishing and neglected scourge of Guinea worm disease.

This disease, which predated the colonial era, had tormented and terrorized Nigerians for 53 years after Nigeria's Independence in 1960, for 28 years after the National Conference on Guinea worm disease, for 27 years after the World Health Assembly passed a resolution for the eradication of the disease and for 25 years after Nigeria signed a memorandum of understanding with The Carter Center for its elimination.

Today, Guinea worm disease is dead, un-mourned, despised and dishonored (without a grave) and it cannot be resuscitated or resurrected! In October 2018, Nigeria should have many justifiable reasons to celebrate that for the last 5 years since independence 58 years ago, the country has been free of Guinea worm disease.

CHAPTER 18

Dracunculiasis Is Gone but Where Is the Pen?

WHERE IS THE PEN?

During the 1992 Opening Ceremony of Nigeria's Annual Commemoration of Guinea Worm Day (every 20th of March), Professor G.L. Monekosso, the Afro-Regional Director of the World Health Organization (WHO), while appreciating Nigeria's aggressive drive toward the elimination of dracunculiasis in the country (under the unparalleled leadership of the late Professor Olikoye Ransome-Kuti, the Hon. Minister of Health), donated a golden pen to sign the obituary of Guinea worm disease at some time in the future when the mission was eventually accomplished (Fig. 18.1).

About two decades later, the transmission of dracunculiasis was successfully interrupted in Nigeria and in 2013, the WHO certified the Federal Republic of Nigeria free of Guinea worm disease! Sadly, Professor Olikoye Ransome-Kuti, the erstwhile Honorable Minister of Health who pioneered the elimination of dracunculiasis in Nigeria, was deceased and Resting in Perfect Peace before Nigeria was certified free of Guinea worm disease.

Today, Guinea worm disease is dead, unburied, unmourned and unresurrectable! As good and fulfilling as this is, the golden pen donated by Professor G.L. Monekosso (the WHO Afra-Regional Director) to sign the obituary of dracunculiasis in Nigeria, has remained missing!

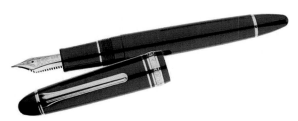

FIG. 18.1 The fountain pen donated by Professor G.L. Monekosso (Afro-Regional Director of WHO) in 1992 to sign the obituary of Guinea worm disease when the disease was eventually eliminated in Nigeria.

The Eradication of Dracunculiasis (Guinea Worm Disease) in Nigeria. https://doi.org/10.1016/B978-0-12-816764-9.00018-3

CHAPTER 19

Counting the Cost and the Scars but the End Justifies the Means!

Dracunculiasis (Guinea worm disease) which had tormented, terrorized, incapacitated, impoverished and stigmatized many Nigerians year after year, pre-dated the colonial era.

Before its eventual elimination and before Nigeria was certified as freed of the disease by the World Health Organization, the water-transmitted parasitic disease had lasted for 53 years after Nigeria's Independence, 28 years after the first National Conference (when the occurrence, magnitude, impact and spread of the disease was first publicly declared in Nigeria), 27 years after the World Health Assembly passed a resolution for its eradication and 25 years after Nigeria signed a Memorandum of Understanding with The Carter Center for its elimination.

The elimination of Guinea worm disease in Nigeria had attracted considerable investments in human and material resources, diplomacy, time, devotion, emotions, sacrifice, perseverance and the worst combination of all the things we dread the most: sickness; discomfort; fear; anxieties; humiliation; separation from loved ones; death; unjustifiable suspicion; injustice; conflict of interests; all shades of deprivation; loss of money and other possessions; ignorance; poverty; neglect; long, stressful, dangerous, and persistent travels; scarcity of vital resources; unlimited exposure to fears and dangers of insecurities, hate, and banditry; very harsh and unfavorable weather; loss of job opportunities; interrupted educational dreams and advancements; unfulfilled, delayed, or missed marriages; blackmail; stigmatization; hazardous exposure to infectious diseases; very deplorable or no access to health care facilities; loss of values and the disappointment of unfulfilled expectations of promises and dreams.

The list is uncountable in number and immeasurable in consequences. Everyone concerned has his/her own share of experiences, hardships and challenges to recount.

The efforts that led to the elimination of Guinea worm disease in Nigeria are equivalent to engaging in war, a fierce battle that lasted for more than 2 decades and left shallow or deep scars of war and victory on many of us. It is equally very gratifying and fulfilling that the fierce battle was tactically fought, gallantly executed and decisively won as evident by the WHO certifying Nigeria free of dracunculiasis in 2013.

It is also gratifying that after the elimination of dracunculiasis in Nigeria, many friends had been made, partnerships strengthened and the euphoria of serving the nation, humanity and the Almighty God had echoed far and wide.

However, the greatest and most enduring fulfillment is that Guinea worm disease and all the woes associated with it have been permanently banished, leaving behind valuable lessons, clues, tools, and experiences that could be successfully used in similar wars against other neglected tropical diseases of medical, socioeconomic and public health significance.

HAS THE END NOT JUSTIFIED THE MEANS?

Personally, on my body, in my flesh and deep down in my soul, I am carrying multiple deep scars of the battle for the elimination of Guinea worm disease with humility, joy, gratitude and a great sense of fulfilment because the end has amply justified the means! (Fig. 19.1A–C).

The Eradication of Dracunculiasis (Guinea Worm Disease) in Nigeria. https://doi.org/10.1016/B978-0-12-816764-9.00019-5

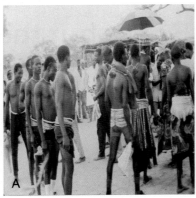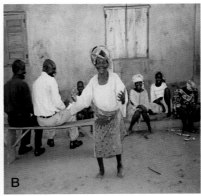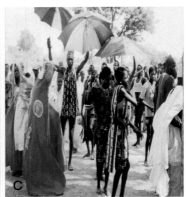

FIG. 19.1 **(A–C)** Celebration of the "obituary" of Guinea worm disease with village traditional dances.

CHAPTER 20

Conclusions

Amidst justifiable skepticism, Nigeria, which at the outset of the eradication drive was the most endemic country in the world (with about 700,000 cases in some 6000 endemic villages, in virtually all States and Local Government Areas [LGAs]), was certified free of Guinea worm disease by the World Health Organization in 2013!

This feat provides good evidence, support, justification, inspiration, encouragement and promise, not only that the ancient dracunculiasis is eradicable but that some other hitherto neglected tropical diseases of significant medical and public health importance can be eradicated, using similar concerted approaches and strategies.

The proven strategies that worked for the successful elimination of Guinea worm disease in Nigeria include: adequate safe water supplies, regular use, and maintenance; uninterrupted and effective health education; vector control using temephos [Abate] and filtration of drinking pond water to sieve out infected cyclops before consumption.

In addition, very good program structures (including multisectoral participation), strong political will and timely action (at Federal, State, LGA, and community levels), robust international support and partnership, good surveillance and effective radical innovations such as surgical extraction of worms, cash rewards, case containment, investigative rumored cases, the use of pond guards, and the provision of incentives (e.g., the Jimmy Carter and Rosalynn Carter Awards, the Guinea Worm Race, etc.), were complementary and enabling strategies effectively used (Fig. 20.1).

As creditable, valuable and indisputable as those intervention strategies were, it must be recognized and admitted that the most powerful, potent and absolutely reliable intervention which, hitherto, has remained unsung, underestimated, ignored and undocumented, is the grace and mercy of the Almighty God!

As mentioned in Chapter 4, the "fiery serpent" which God used to punish the grumbling Israelites in the wilderness during their mass exodus away from slavery in Egypt, was actually Guinea worm disease. Alfred J. Bollett, a Professor of clinical medicine at Yale University School of Medicine was strongly persuasive that the Biblical "fiery serpents" were indeed Guinea worms.[1] He is the same God, who, at this point in time, has mercifully, graciously and miraculously made the elimination of our endemic dracunculiasis possible.

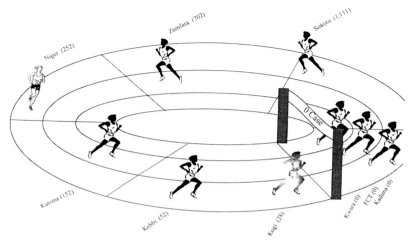

FIG. 20.1 The Guinea worm Race in the North West Zone of NIGEP by State (January - December, 2000).

Thus, an analogy can be made that:

- Currently, in our own situation, the "fiery serpent" remains the same Guinea worm;
- "The bronze serpent" on the pole is the intervention we applied to eliminate the disease and
- Moses (the Prophet) is symbolically the Jimmy Carters, the Yakubu Gowons, the Richard Reids, the Olikoye Ransome-Kutis, the Don Hopkins, the leaders of United Nations, Non-government Organization, Governments and all those who participated actively at all levels.

When we seek God's interventions in our individual, collective, local, national and global affairs, including for the control/eradication of dracunculiasis and other tropical challenges, God's grace, compassion, and mercy endure forever. With Him, nothing is impossible! God is still the same, omnipotent.

Unlike the skepticism expressed before the miraculous elimination of dracunculiasis in Nigeria (I was an eyewitness of some of those verifiable circumstances), we cannot and should not be skeptical about what the Almighty God can do!

REFERENCE

1. Hopkins DR, Hopkins EM. *Guinea worm: The End in Sight. Encyclopedia Britannica.* Chicago: Medical and Health Annual; 1992:10—27.

Key Stakeholders/Partners Involved in the Elimination of Dracunculiasis in Nigeria

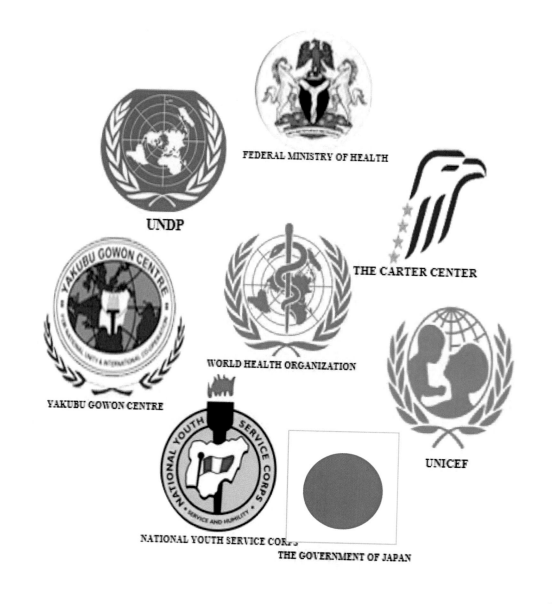

FEDERAL MINISTRY OF HEALTH

UNDP

THE CARTER CENTER

WORLD HEALTH ORGANIZATION

YAKUBU GOWON CENTRE

NATIONAL YOUTH SERVICE CORPS

THE GOVERNMENT OF JAPAN

UNICEF

1. Logos of some key stakeholders/partners involved in the elimination of dracunculiasis in Nigeria
2. Nigeria Guinea worm commemorative postage stamps
3. Some memorable notes on dracunculiasis
4. The Guinea worm race in the NIGEP North West Zone (January - December, 2000)
5. Some notable photographs of Guinea worm disease during elimination activities in Nigeria
6. Quotable quotes on Guinea worm disease

Nigeria Guinea Worm Commemorative Postage Stamps

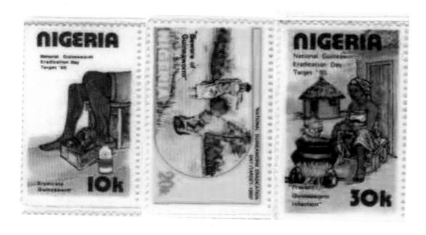

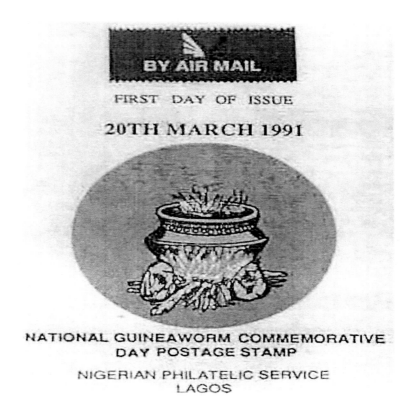

Some Memorable Notes on Dracunculiasis from Friends/Colleagues

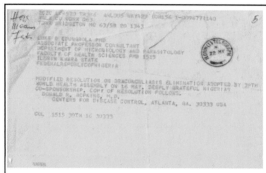

LUKE D. EDUNGBOLA PHD
ASSOCIATE PROFESSOR CONSULTANT
DEPARTMENT OF MICROBIOLOGY AND PARASITOLOGY
FACULTY OF HEALTH SCIENCES PMB 1515
ILORIN KWARA STATE
FEDERAL REPUBLIC OF NIGERIA

MODIFIED RESOLUTION ON DRACUNCULIASIS ELIMINATION ADOPTED BY 39TH WORLD HEALTH ASSEMBLY ON 16TH MAY. DEEPLY GRATEFUL NIGERIAN CO-SPONSORSHIP. COPY OF RESOLUTION FOLLOWS.
  DONALD R. HOPKINS, M.D.
    CENTER FOR DISEASE CONTROL, ATLANTA, GA. 30333 USA

A

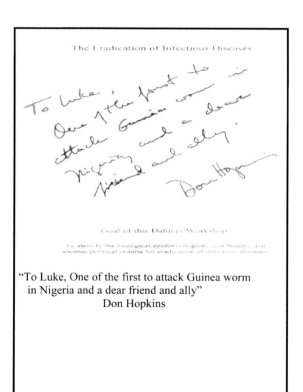

"To Luke, One of the first to attack Guinea worm
  in Nigeria and a dear friend and ally"
        Don Hopkins

B

"Luke, Good job !
Give each zonal consultant a copy of your complete line list <u>now.</u>
    Ask them to:
  (1) verify
  (2) add number of <u>functioning</u> safe sources there (whether from 2002 or earlier)
  (3) note whether water supply in each village is <u>adequate</u> or not"

C

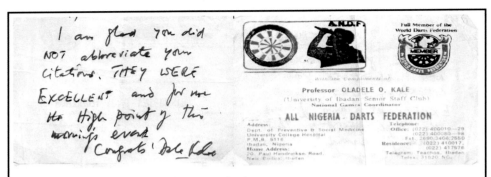

"I am glad you did NOT abbreviate your citations.
THEY WERE EXCELLENT and for me the High Point
of this morning's event
Congrats ! Dele Kale"

D

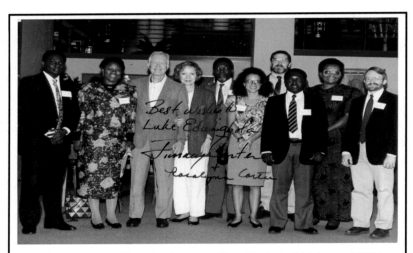

President Jimmy and Rosalyn Carter and Two Technical Advisers of TCC in Photograph with the Nigerian delegates to the Ghana-Nigeria GWD Programme Review at The Carter Center in Atlanta, GA, USA in 1991.

E

The Guinea Worm Race
January—December (2000)

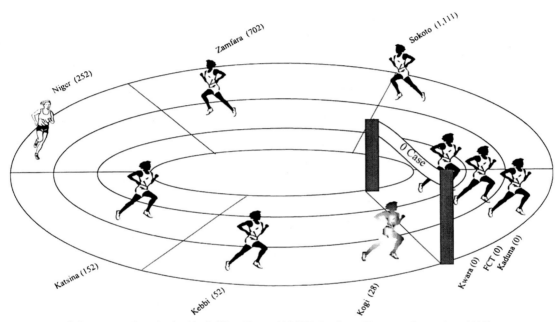

Guinea worm Race in the North West Zone of NIGEP, by State (January—December, 2000)

Some Notable Photographs of Guinea Worm Disease During Elimination Activities in Nigeria

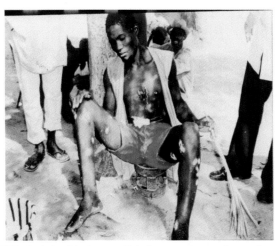

FIG. 1 A terribly incapacitated young farmer from whose body a world record of 84 Guinea worms were extracted in a single transmission year.

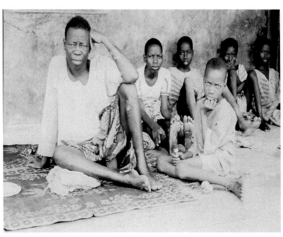

FIG. 2 A successful Lagos-based business man was returned to the village with the emergence of multiple Guinea worms on his legs and left arm. His five children are seen with him, also incapacitated with multiple infections and could not go to school.

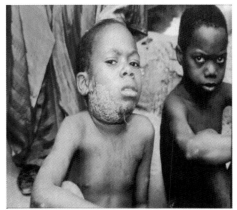

FIG. 3 Two infected primary school boys. The boy on the left has Guinea worm emerging from his badly swollen jaw, a very dangerous location, being close to the brain.

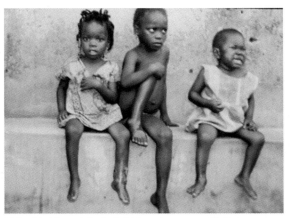

FIG. 4A Three infected children in agony with Guinea worm disease on their feet.

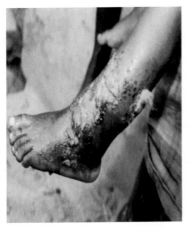

FIG. 4B The badly infected left leg of the first girl from the left. (In Fig. 4A)

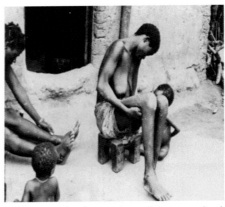

FIG. 5A Two nursing housewives of the same husband in agony with dracunculiasis, leaving their infants neglected and poorly cared for.

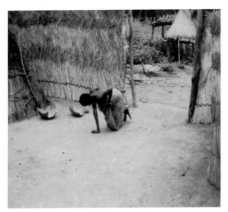

FIG. 5B The woman on the right (in Fig. 5A) was just returning (crawling on her knees) from the backyard to relieve herself.

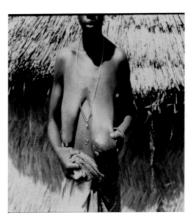

FIG. 5C The same woman, 2 weeks later with her left mammary gland becoming a fibrotic mass and producing no milk to feed the baby in a most rural setting where and when no marketed baby food was available. The babies became badly malnourished.

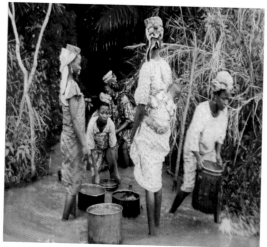

FIG. 6 Housewives ignorantly wading into this pond and contaminating it. At least two of them had emerging Guinea worms on their legs.

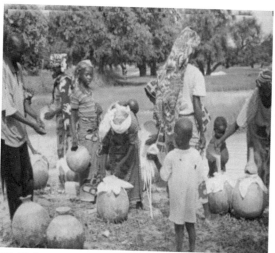

FIG. 7 One of the most effective radical innovations in the North West Zone was the placement of good and sufficient filters, bowls, buckets and a pond guard at unsafe water collection sites to encourage and ensure that the water fetched for drinking was filtered even before taking the water home.

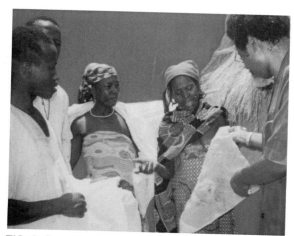

FIG. 8 One of the four core NIGEP intervention strategies in the elimination of Guinea worm disease: regular filter inspection, replacement, correct usage and availability to all households.

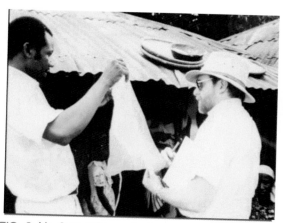

FIG. 9 Mr. Craig Withers, Jr. (Director of Operation, TCC) and the Niger State Guinea worm Coordinator jointly examining the condition of a household filter.

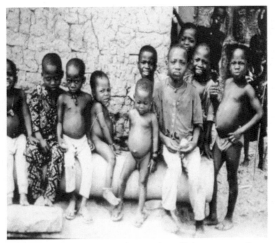

FIG. 10 Traditional protection against Guinea worm disease being worn on the hands, legs and around the necks of children in an hyperendemic village: a perceived form of native intervention.

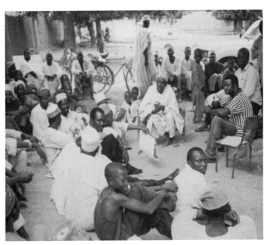

FIG. 11 Massive health education in Tsogawa, Kankia Local Government Areas, Kastina State, following an outbreak and just before large-scale surgical extraction of Guinea worms. Solomon Olukade, a most celebrated Nigerian in surgical extraction of Guinea worms, is in white and black stripes, sitting close to the Village Head.

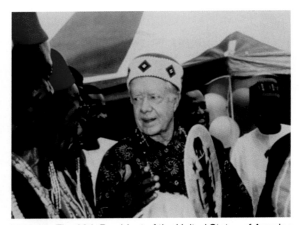

FIG. 12 The 39th President of the United States of America and Chairman of The Carter Center is being traditionally decorated in appreciation of his role in dracunculiasis elimination in Nigeria.

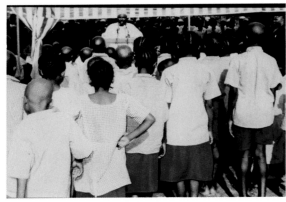

FIG. 13A During his advocacy and intervention activities to endemic areas, Gen. Dr. Yakubu Gowon was giving health education to school children.

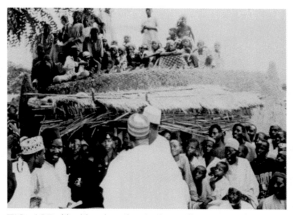

FIG. 13B Health education to the entire community, some climbing on the thatched rooftop to see and hear Gen. Gowon. The Chairman of Bukuyum LGA is seen on the left, facing the camera and smiling.

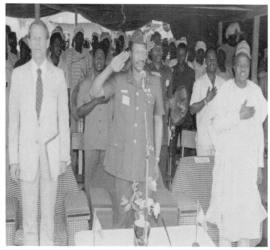

FIG. 14 Opening ceremony of the 1985 First National Conference on Guinea Worm Disease in Nigeria (Left to right): Mr. Richard Reid (UNICEF Country Representative in Nigeria); Group Captain Salaudeen Adebola Latinwo (Military Governor of Kwara State) and Alh. Adamu Gene (Hon. Commissioner for Local Government and Cheiftaincy Affairs).

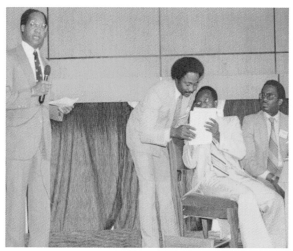

FIG. 15 First National Dracunculiasis Conference in Ilorin, Kwara State, Nigeria (1985). Left to right: Dr. Donald R. Hopkins, Centers for Disease Control and Prevention/Global 2000 making his presentation; the late Dr. Yinka Ajayi Dopemu sharing conference information with Dr. Luke Edungbola (the convener) as Professor Pekun Alausa listened to Dr. Hopkins' presentation.

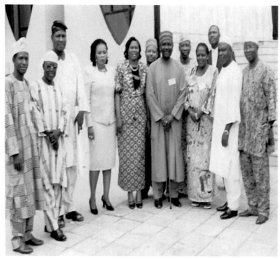

FIG. 16 The NIGEP/The Carter Center Participants at the International Regional Meeting on Dracunculiasis. Gen. Dr. Yakubu Gowon is seen in the center. The late Dr. K.A. Ojudu (the NIGEP National Coordinator, 1995–2007) is on the extreme right. Next to Ojudu, in white dress, is Dr. E.S. Miri, The Carter Center Country Representative (Nigeria).

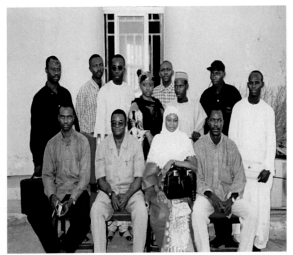

FIG. 17 NIGEP/The Carter Center field staff based in Katsina State.

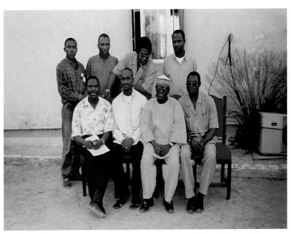

FIG. 18 Some Senior Staff of NIGEP/The Carter Center, North West Zone, based in the Secretariat from where they serve all the 9 States in the zone.

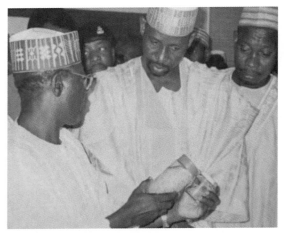

FIG. 19 The Carter Center Senior Zonal Consultants (left) showing specimen bottles full of extracted Guinea worms to the Deputy Governor of Zamfara State at the exhibition desk during a Zonal Task Force Meeting in Gusau.

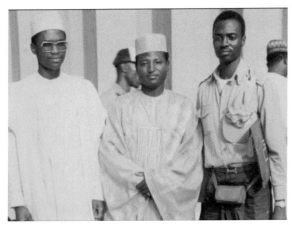

FIG. 20 Presentation of President Jimmy Carter and Rosalynn Carter awards at an Annual Guinea Worm Day (March 20). All the winners for the year were from the North West Zone. Left to right: Bello Dogondaji (Sokoto State Guinea worm Coordinator) won Second prize; Alh Danjuma Baba (Executive Chairman Paiko LGA) won the First prize, and Baba Ahmed (the first Youth Corps Member to serve in the North West Zone and who served for more than 2 decades until Guinea worm disease was eliminated in Nigeria), won the Third prize.

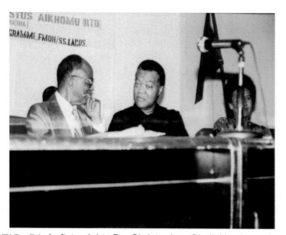

FIG. 21 Left to right: Dr. Christopher Okoji (the incoming Minister of Health), Professor Olikoye Ransome-Kuti (Minister of Health) and Mrs. Olikoye Ransome-Kuti on the High Table during the launching of the Guinea worm Commemorative Postage Stamp.

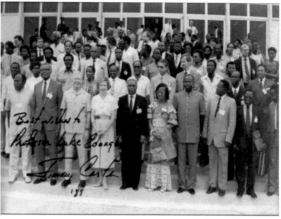

FIG. 22 Second African Regional Meeting on Dracunculiasis was held in Accra, Ghana, in 1988 during when the universal definition of a case of Guinea worm disease was established. Center: Professor and Mrs. G.I. Monekosso (Director of the WHO Afro Regional Office); President Jimmy and Rosalynn Carter on the right of Professor Monekosso and to the left of Mrs. Monekesso is Professor A.B.C. Nwosu, Nigeria's Hon. Minister of Health and the first to launch a State Guinea worm Task Force in Nigeria.

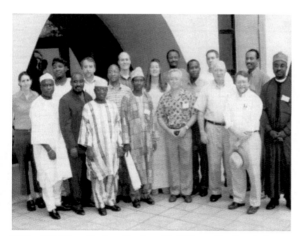

FIG. 23 The Carter Center Staff/Consultants during a Regional Meeting on Guinea worm disease in Lome, Togo.

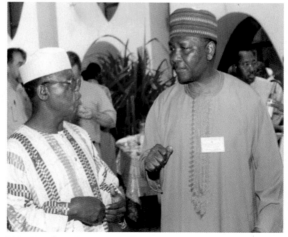

FIG. 24 Gen. Dr. Yakubu Gowon (former Head of State and Chairman, the Yakubu Gowon Centre) in a discussion with Professor Luke Edungbola on dracunculiasis elimination in Nigeria.

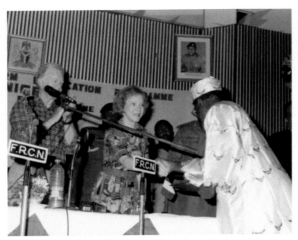

FIG. 25 President Jimmy and Rosalynn Carter presenting the Merit Award to Professor Luke Edungbola for his outstanding contributions to dracunculiasis elimination in Nigeria.

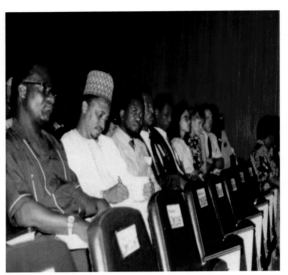

FIG. 26 Participants at the Donors' Conference on Dracunculiasis.

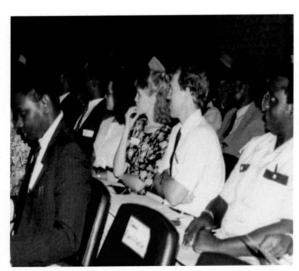

FIG. 27 American Medical Students' Association Fellows (AMSA) at the Donors' Conference. From the right: the late Dr. J.O. Idowu, Director of the Epidemiology Unit; Chris Crosdale and his AMSA colleagues.

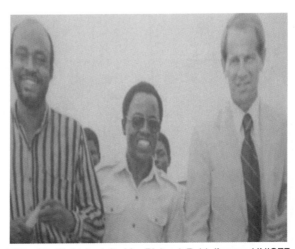

FIG. 28 Right to left: Mr. Richard Reid (former UNICEF Country Representative in Nigeria) was one of the earliest and most outstanding sponsors, motivators, and supporters of dracunculiasis elimination in Nigeria; Dr. Luke Edungbola (College of Health Sciences, University of Ilorin, Ilorin); and Mr. Sule Garba, first Coordinator of UNICEF Programs in Kwara State.

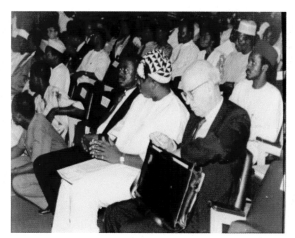

FIG. 29 The Third Guinea Worm Disease Day (March 20). In white spotted traditional cap is Professor A.B.C. Nwosu (Minister of Health) and the former American Ambassador to Nigeria, Ambassador Easum, is sitting on the left of Professor A.B.C Nwosu.

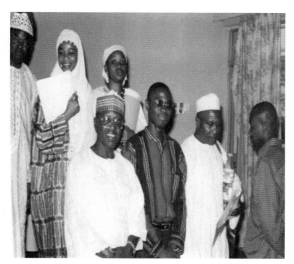

FIG. 31 Some members of staff of NIGEP/The Carter Center, North West Zone, during the National Programme Review. Dr. E.S. Miri, The Carter Center Country Representative, is in the traditional white cap.

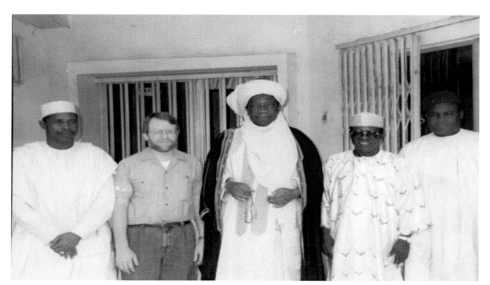

FIG. 30 General Sani Same (retired), the Emir of Zuru (center); Craig Withers Jr. (Director of Operations, The Carter Center, Atlanta, GA, USA) is on the right of the Emir and Professor Luke Edungbola (Senior Consultant NIGEP/The Carter Center, is on the left of the Emir. The Director of Primary Health Care (Zuru LGA) and the Secretary to the Emir, are on the extreme left and right, respectively.

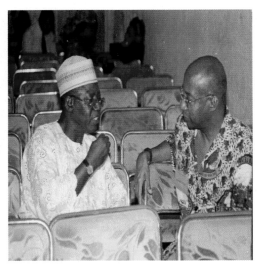

FIG. 32 Dr. Donald R. Hopkins (Vice-President and Director of the Health Program, The Carter Center, in a heart to heart discussion on dracunculiasis elimination with Professor Luke D. Edungbola, The Carter Center National Technical Adviser.

Some Quotable Quotes on Guinea Worm Disease

Once you've seen a small child with a two-foot-long live Guinea worm protruding from her body, right through a large sore between her toes, you never forget it.

PRESIDENT JIMMY CARTER (THE 39TH PRESIDENT OF THE UNITED STATES AND CHAIRMAN OF THE CARTER CENTER).

A reporter in Africa once asked me, "Why in the world are you involved in a program to eliminate Guinea worm disease?" The answer is easy. There is no reason people should suffer from an affliction that is so easy to prevent.

PRESIDENT JIMMY CARTER (FORMER PRESIDENT OF USA).

Your choice of Ilorin, the Kwara State capital, as the venue for this first ever conference on dracunculiasis is not only because of the reported existence of Guinea worm in the State, but rather, in recognition of the positive efforts of the State Government in the areas of eradication and control of Guinea worm and other water-borne diseases in the State.

GROUP CAPTAIN S.A. LATINWO (MILITARY GOVERNOR OF KWARA STATE) AT THE FIRST NATIONAL GUINEA WORM CONFERENCE IN ILORIN, 1985.

This is a historic occasion and a historic location. Fifteen years ago, only a few kilometers outside Ilorin, the last case of smallpox in West Africa occurred. It is thus especially fitting that this meeting, which begins the public campaign to eradicate another disease in Africa, should be convened in this time and place.

DONALD R. HOPKINS (DEPUTY DIRECTOR, CDC, ATLANTA GEORGIA, USA) AT THE FIRST NATIONAL GUINEA WORM CONFERENCE IN ILORIN, 1985.

I understand that this conference is the foundation of the commitment which will pave way for the eradication of Guinea worm disease in Nigeria and elsewhere in Africa.

GROUP CAPTAIN S.A. LATINWO (MILITARY GOVERNOR OF KWARA STATE) AT THE FIRST NATIONAL GUINEA WORM CONFERENCE IN ILORIN, 1985.

These Nigerian "firsts" are a valuable example to other African countries with Guinea worm: the first national case search in Africa; the first National Guinea Worm Conference; the first national policy of priority for water supply to villages with Guinea worm; and the first commemorative postage stamps.

DONALD R. HOPKINS (SENIOR CONSULTANT, GLOBAL 2000).

Guinea worm disease is an avoidable suffering of an unnecessary cause and the cause of an unnecessary suffering. Its eradication is an equivalent of a war which must be disseminated to all nations and peoples: When there is no time, Guinea worm disease should be mentioned first; when there is little time, Guinea worm disease should be mentioned first and last; and when there is more time, Guinea worm disease should be mentioned again and again.

PROFESSOR LUKE D. EDUNGBOLA.

This conference on dracunculiasis eradication is spectacular. If Guinea worm disease has a pair of boots, it will be shaking in them.

DONALD R. HOPKINS (SENIOR CONSULTANT, GLOBAL 2000).

The conference has made some far-reaching recommendations and it is our hope that those who are in a position to act on them would do so as a matter of urgency. Think of all those millions of Nigerians who would benefit when this serious public problem is eradicated and think of the benefits which will accrue to the entire nation through better health for many of its citizens and increased agricultural production. We cannot afford to wait any longer.

PROFESSOR UMARU SHEHU, FAS (WHO REPRESENTATIVE, NIGERIA).

Distinguished guests, Guinea worm does not have a right to exist in our midst, it must be eradicated. All hands must be on deck, because Guinea worm is not just a health problem, it is also an agriculture, socio-economic, and educational problem. It is a problem that relates to the dignity, pride, and fundamental human right of mankind. It is a problem not only for the Federal Government but also for the States, Local Government and, indeed, all citizens of the entire nation. This time, we should not and must not relent in our efforts. We should make the life of our children and future generation of Nigeria better than our own.

PROFESSOR OLIKOYE RANSOME-KUTI (HON. MINISTER OF HEALTH).

It is because of the seriousness of this disease that during the National Council of Health held in Abuja last year, it was approved that Guinea worm disease be made a notifiable disease in Nigeria.

PROFESSOR OLIKOYE RANSOME-KUTI (HON. MINISTER OF HEALTH).

To make 1995 a reality, my Ministry has set up a National Task Force on Guinea Worm Eradication and all the States have done the same. The Nigeria Guinea Worm Eradication Programme (NIGEP) Secretariat has been established in the Department of Disease Control and International Health of my Ministry and has the responsibilities of nationwide co-ordination of the guinea worm program.

PROFESSOR OLIKOYE RANSOME-KUTI (HON. MINISTER OF HEALTH).

Guinea worm disease is the first and potentially feasible disease to be eradicated without using drug or vaccine. I will conclude by regarding this gathering as a religious congregation with a common faith, a common commitment, and a common hope. The common faith is that Guinea worm, which is widespread and highly prevalent in Nigeria, can be eliminated within the available resources at the nation's disposal. Our common commitment is to eliminate Guinea worm in Nigeria and elsewhere and the hope is that it will be done.

PROFESSOR LUKE D. EDUNGBOLA.

We announce today that DFRRI will now use the presence of Guinea worm disease as the primary criterion for targeting water supply, such as hand-dug wells and boreholes. Villages with Guinea worm will now be a priority for all water supply projects in Nigeria (including UNICEF and UNDP/World Bank water projects). The attack phase will require a greater commitment on the part of everyone involved.

VICE-ADMIRAL AUGUSTUS AIKHOMU (CHIEF OF GENERAL STAFF).

Therefore, elimination of Guinea worm makes economic as well as moral sense.

KRISTIAN LAUBJERG (UNICEF REPRESENTATIVE TO NIGERIA).

The efforts to which we are all contributing to today should not be relaxed until we have achieved the primary objective of this meeting — to eradicate dracunculiasis as an unnecessary cause of misery, agony, and poverty, so that our people may live better and longer, particularly for Nigeria and for humanity in general.

PROFESSOR LUKE D. EDUNGBOLA.

Moreover, the National Council on Health declared Guinea worm to be an officially reportable disease, and established the national goal of eradicating dracunculiasis from Nigeria by 1995. More astonishingly, you have carried out, in the face of many who doubted you could or would do it, a nationwide search for cases which reached into almost every village of this vast country. The way you accomplished this first search will be long remembered in the annals of international public health.

DONALD R. HOPKINS (SENIOR CONSULTANT, GLOBAL 2000).

The simple answer is to ask, "If Nigeria can do it, and they have the most Guinea worm, what's your excuse?" This is a war, not a tea party. People are suffering, we already know how to help them. We cannot shorten the one year incubation period of this disease, each delay of a few weeks can mean another whole year of suffering for some. We must act now!

DONALD R. HOPKINS (SENIOR CONSULTANT, GLOBAL 2000).

It must be borne in mind that the tragedy in life doesn't lie in not reaching your goal, the tragedy lies in having no goal to reach. It isn't a calamity to die with dreams unfulfilled, but it is a calamity not to dream. It is not a disaster to be unable to capture your ideal, but it is a disaster to have no ideal to capture. It is not a disgrace not to reach the stars, but it is a disgrace to have no stars to reach for. Not failure, but low aim is a sin.

DR. BENJAMIN ELIJAH MAYS (PRESIDENT OF MOREHOUSE COLLEGE) QUOTED BY DR. D.R. HOPKINS.

Although a variety of cultural, traditional, and scientific approaches have been used over the years to deal with Guinea worm disease, the fact remains that the best strategy to eliminate it completely is by providing safe drinking water, since Guinea worm disease is transmitted exclusively by drinking contaminated water.

PROFESSOR S. AFOLABI-TOYE (VICE-CHANCELLOR, UNIVERSITY OF ILORIN IN 1985).

Guinea worm knows no boundaries, national or international. UNICEF has therefore established a special unit in New York and has appointed a coordinator for the Guinea worm eradication effort in Africa. It is not by chance that the coordinator is based in Nigeria. Since Nigeria has 60% of the world's cases, it can and must lead the worldwide effort to eliminate this parasite.

KRISTIAN LAUBJERG (UNICEF REPRESENTATIVE TO NIGERIA).

Dracunculiasis is a disease that opens itself for eradication. The WHO has committed itself to this goal by the year 1995. Africa, which is the continent currently with the highest number of cases and population at risk, stands to gain in the areas of health, agriculture, education and general socio-economic development if this disease is eradicated on schedule.

DR. S.H. BREW-GRAVES (WHO REPRESENTATIVE TO NIGERIA).

I am particularly appreciative of the work of the Nigeria Guinea Worm Eradication Task Force, as I come from one of the parts of the country — Anambra State — where the endemicity of the disease is high and where the award winning film, The Fiery Serpent, was shot.

PROFESSOR GORDIAN EZEKWE (HON. MINISTER OF SCIENCE AND TECHNOLOGY).

I wish to state that our support of the work of both Professor A.B.C. Nwosu of the University of Nigeria, Nsukka, who is now Anambra State Commissioner of Health, and that of Professor Edungbola of the University of Ilorin, went a long way to awakening the conscience of the nation to address the Guinea worm problem.

PROFESSOR GORDIAN EZEKWE (HON. MINISTER OF SCIENCE AND TECHNOLOGY).

In the awareness campaign to eradicate the Guinea worm disease, the Nigerian Postal Service Department (NIPOST) is today releasing a set of special postage stamps in the denominations of 10 kobo, 20 kobo, and 30 kobo.

ENGR. OLAWALE IGE (HON. MINISTER OF COMMUNICATIONS).

Since the ultimate goal of our Guinea worm eradication efforts is the provision of potable drinking water, efforts will be made to allocate more resources to DFRRI to ensure that water points are provided to the 6000 endemic Guinea worm villages. I wish to also appeal to international water agencies to move to the remote, hard to reach, rural, and most important, Guinea worm endemic villages with their water programs. For effective implementation of the program, emphasis has now been shifted to the 6000 Guinea worm affected villages which are the direct responsibility of the local government. As the saying goes "Charity begins at home". To this end, I wish to announce that Local Government Chairman in Guinea worm endemic areas should allocate at least 10% of their health project to Guinea worm eradication activities.

ADMIRAL AUGUSTUS AIKHOMU (VICE-PRESIDENT, FEDERAL REPUBLIC OF NIGERIA).

Nigeria is the greatest beneficiary worldwide from the donation of both nylon filter material and Abate. NIGEP is leaving no stone unturned to maximize the benefits that will accrue from their use.

PROFESSOR OLADELE O. KALE (NATIONAL CHAIRMAN, NIGEP/NATIONAL TASK FORCE).

Index

Note: Page numbers followed by "f" indicate figures, "t" indicate tables.

Printed in the United States
By Bookmasters